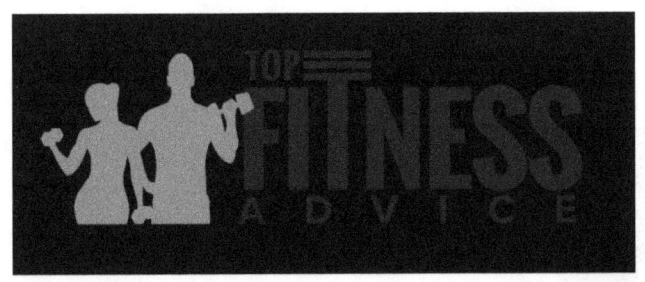

DASH DIET

2nd Edition

The DASH Diet for Beginners – DASH Diet Quick Start Guide with 35 FAT-BLASTING Tips & 21 Quick & Tasty Recipes That Will Lower YOUR Blood Pressure!

LINDA WESTWOOD

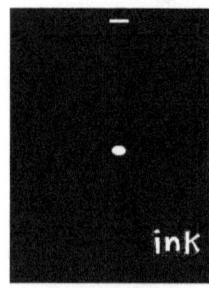

First published in 2015 by Venture Ink Publishing

Copyright © Top Fitness Advice 2019

All rights reserved.

No part of this book may be reproduced in any form without permission in writing from the author. No part of this publication may be reproduced or transmitted in any form or by any means, mechanic, electronic, photocopying, recording, by any storage or retrieval system, or transmitted by email without the permission in writing from the author and publisher.

Requests to the publisher for permission should be addressed to publishing@ventureink.co

For more information about the contents of this book or questions to the author, please contact Linda Westwood at linda@topfitnessadvice.com

Disclaimer

This book provides wellness management information in an informative and educational manner only, with information that is general in nature and that is not specific to you, the reader. The contents of this book are intended to assist you and other readers in your personal wellness efforts. Consult your physician regarding the applicability of any information provided in this book to you.

Nothing in this book should be construed as personal advice or diagnosis, and must not be used in this manner. The information provided about conditions is general in nature. This information does not cover all possible uses, actions, precautions, side-effects, or interactions of medicines, or medical procedures. The information in this book should not be considered as complete and does not cover all diseases, ailments, physical conditions, or their treatment.

You should consult with your physician before beginning any exercise, weight loss, or health care program. This book should not be used in place of a call or visit to a competent health-care professional. You should consult a health care professional before adopting any of the suggestions in this book or before drawing inferences from it.

Any decision regarding treatment and medication for your condition should be made with the advice and consultation of a qualified health care professional. If you have, or suspect you have, a health-care problem, then you should immediately contact a qualified health care professional for treatment.

No Warranties: The author and publisher don't guarantee or warrant the quality, accuracy, completeness, timeliness, appropriateness or suitability of the information in this book, or of any product or services referenced in this book.

The information in this book is provided on an "as is" basis and the author and publisher make no representations or warranties of any kind with respect to this information. This book may contain inaccuracies, typographical errors, or other errors.

Liability Disclaimer: The publisher, author, and other parties involved in the creation, production, provision of information, or delivery of this book specifically disclaim any responsibility, and shall not be held liable for any damages, claims, injuries, losses, liabilities, costs, or obligations including any direct, indirect, special, incidental, or consequences damages (collectively known as "Damages") whatsoever and howsoever caused, arising out of, or in connection with the use or misuse of the site and the information contained within it, whether such Damages arise in contract, tort, negligence, equity, statute law, or by way of other legal theory.

Table of Contents

Disclaimer	3
What will this book teach you?	7
Introduction	9
Meal Plan: Day 1	13
Meal Plan: Day 2	21
Meal Plan: Day 3	31
Meal Plan: Day 4	39
Meal Plan: Day 5	49
Meal Plan: Day 6	59
Meal Plan: Day 7	71
35 Fat-Blasting Tips	81
Final Words	101

Would you prefer to listen to my book, rather than read it?

Download the audiobook version for free!

If you go to the special link below and sign up to Audible as a new customer, you can get the audiobook version of my book completely free.

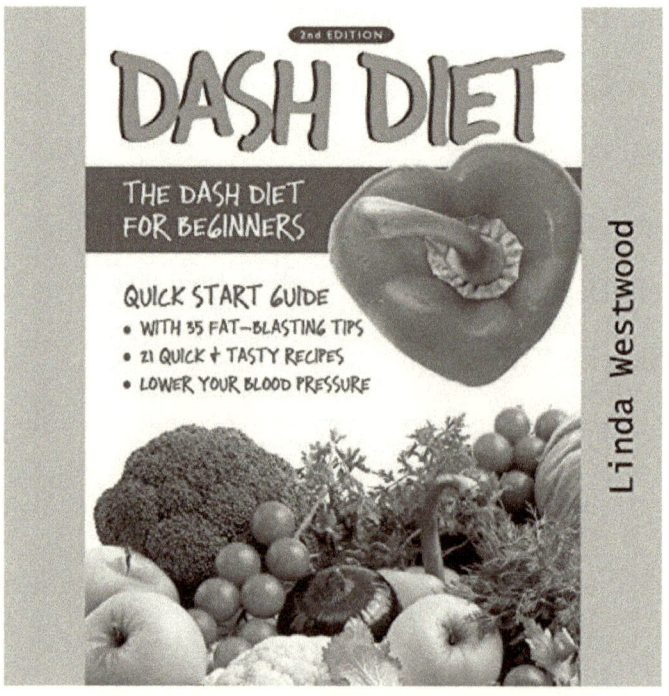

Go here to get your audiobook version for free:

TopFitnessAdvice.com/go/dash

What will this book teach you?

Hypertension and obesity are the biggest issues of our generation. For those of you who are looking to control your hypertension and lose weight at the same time – you can benefit immensely if you follow the tips mentioned in this book.

The most important thing that this book teaches is the fact that being healthy is a **choice** and you can stay healthy by **making the right lifestyle choices**.

The tips mentioned in this book will help you stay fit and maintain an optimal weight and also keep your hypertension under check.

Introduction

DASH stands for Dietary Approaches to Stop Hypertension and thus the DASH diet is primarily designed to help people lower their blood pressure by simply regulating the meals they consume.

Whilst the main purpose of the DASH diet is to aid in regulation of blood pressure, it also turns out to be handy for weight loss.

Here, in this book, we are going to offer you a 7-day DASH diet plan which will help tremendously to ensure that you can keep your blood pressure levels in check, and also lose weight.

The DASH diet is so designed that your body will succeed in attaining the requisite calorie requirements.

The book is structured so that the first section contains the 7-day meal plan, and after this section is the 35 POWERFUL tips to fast track your DASH diet success!

Discover Scientifically-Proven "Shortcuts" & "Hacks" to Lose Weight FASTER (With Very Little Effort)

For this month only, you can get Linda's best-selling & most popular book absolutely free – *Weight Loss Secrets You NEED to Know*.

Get Your FREE Copy Here:
TopFitnessAdvice.com/Bonus

Discover scientifically-proven tips to help you lose weight faster and easier than ever before. With this book, readers were able to improve their weight loss results and fitness levels. So, it's highly recommended that you get this book, especially while it's free!

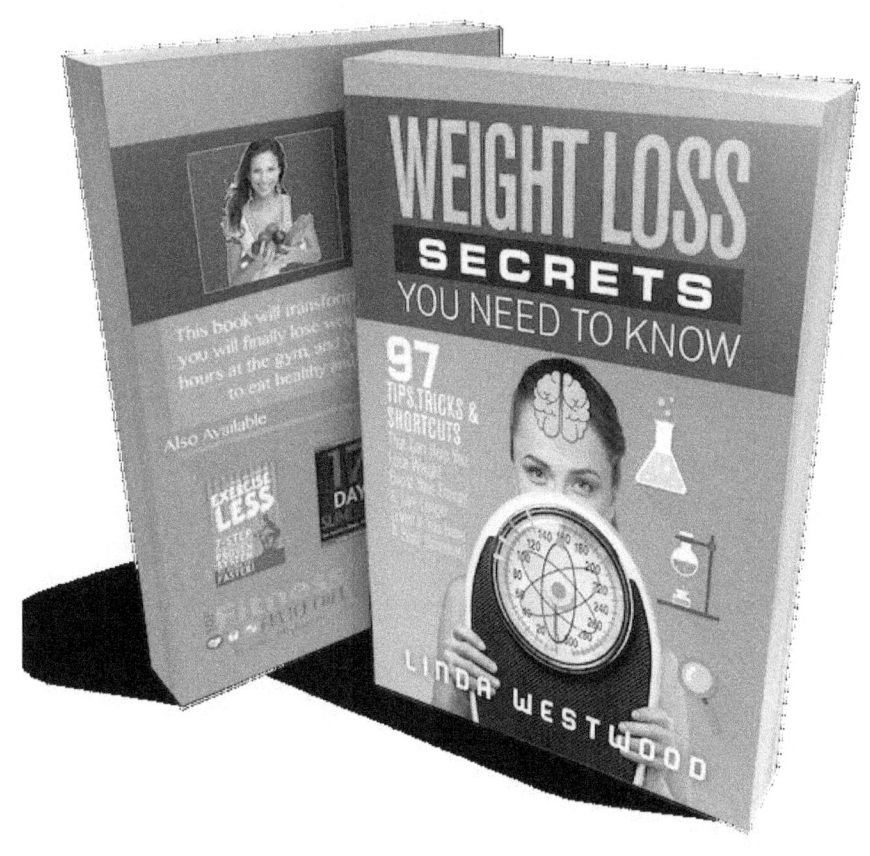

Get Your FREE Copy Here:

TopFitnessAdvice.com/Bonus

Meal Plan

Day 1

Every day, you have to follow the perfect meal plan to keep your sodium levels in check. The overall meal for the day needs to be a mix of proteins, carbohydrates, necessary fats, minerals, vitamins and more.

We will offer you the meal plan for the day by listing the meals you need to have during your breakfast, lunch and dinner.

Breakfast

For your breakfast, you can have the following meals, as it will give you the right energy needed to start your day. Following are the three things you can have for your breakfast.

1. Bran flakes cereal (3/4th cup) - These are a ready-to-eat cereal. You are best advised to have 1 medium banana along with a cup of low-fat milk. This whole meal contains a net sodium count of 328 mg.

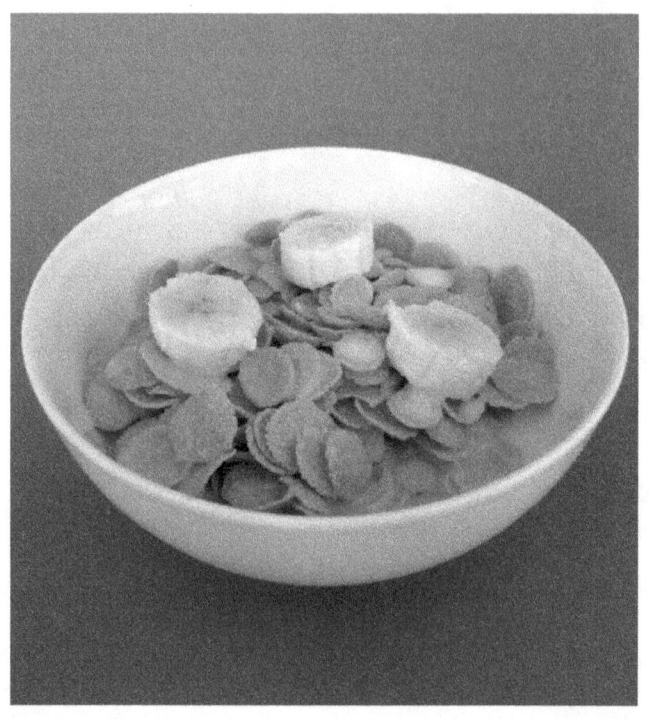

2. A slice of whole wheat bread. Make it a point to use a teaspoon of soft tub margarine.

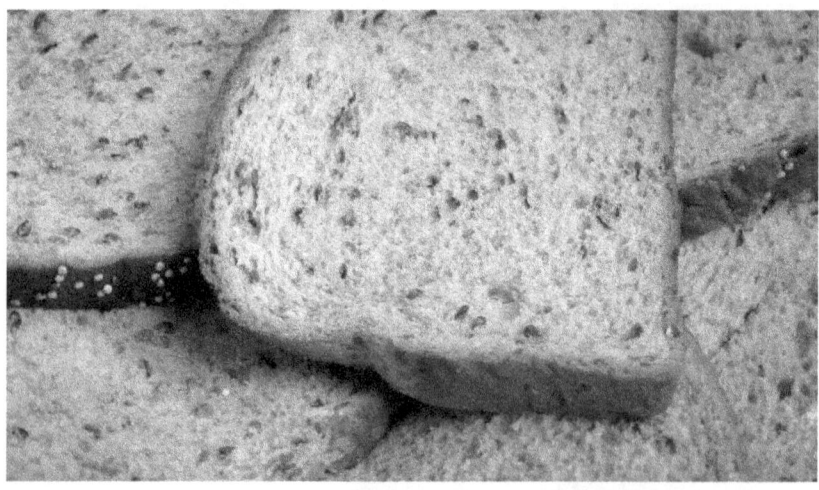

3. To complete your breakfast, add a cup or orange juice. This will add the much-needed fruit to your meal and thereby help you have a complete breakfast.

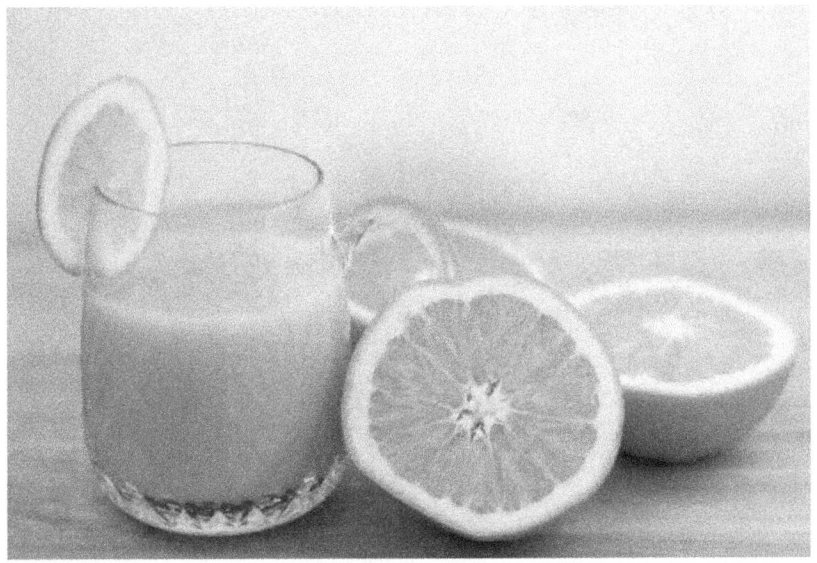

The total sodium count of the whole meal would be below 508 mg.

Lunch

The lunch for your DASH diet day 1 will be a chicken salad.

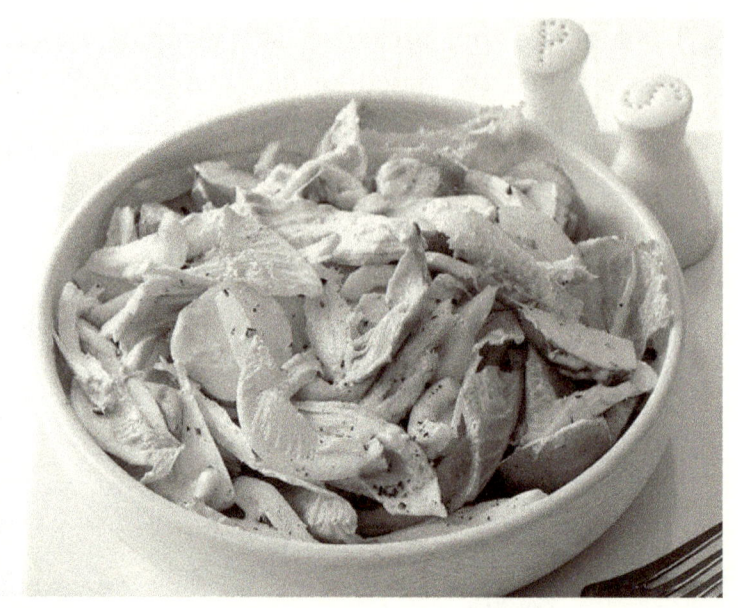

Ingredients

- 3 ¼ cups of chicken that is cooked, cubed and skinless
- 1 tablespoon of lemon juice
- 1/8 teaspoon of salt
- ¼ cup of chopped celery
- ½ teaspoon of onion powder
- 3 tablespoons of low-fat mayonnaise

Instructions

1. Bake the chicken thoroughly. Cut it into cubes and refrigerate it. Take a large bowl and mix all the remaining ingredients in it.

2. Now add the chicken cubes from the refrigerator and mix it well. The dish is ready to be served.

Tip

You can omit 1/8 teaspoon of salt, if you want to cut down your sodium intake even more.

Along with the chicken salad, following are the other side dishes you can have with it to have a complete lunch.

1. A couple of slices of whole wheat bread.

2. ½ cup of fruit cocktail

3. 1 tablespoon of Dijon mustard salad.

Dinner

For your dinner, following are the different meals you can have.

1. Take a 3 oz beef, eye of the round. For the best taste, make sure to add 2 tablespoon of fat free beef gravy.

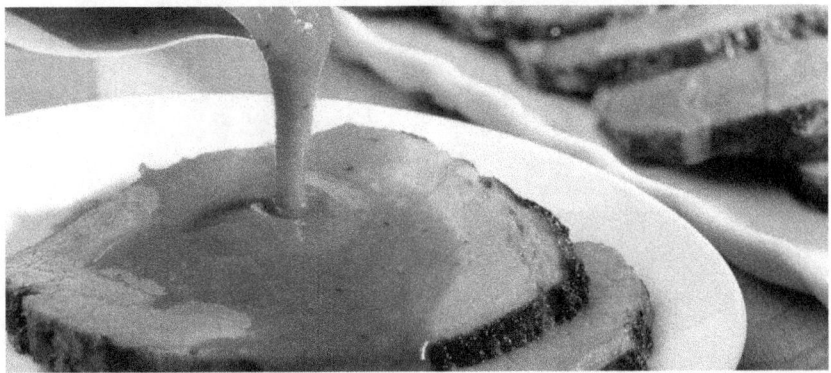

2. 1 baked potato that is small in size. You will need 1 tablespoon of fat free sour cream along with a tablespoon of reduced fat, natural grated cheddar cheese. Finally, use another tablespoon of chopped scallions.

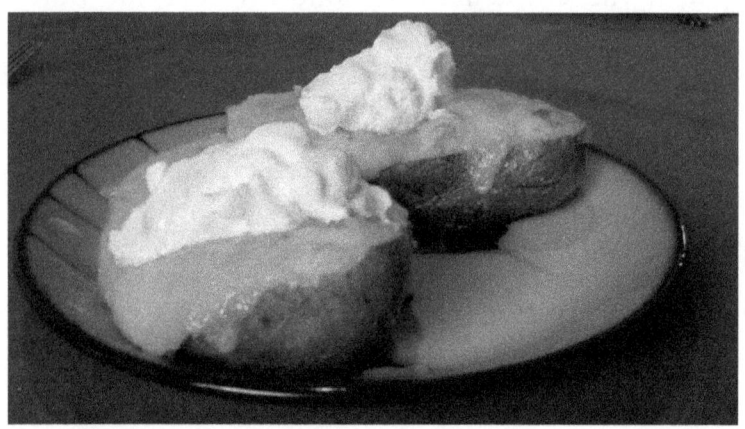

3. Take a cup of green beans that has been sautéed with ½ teaspoon canola oil.

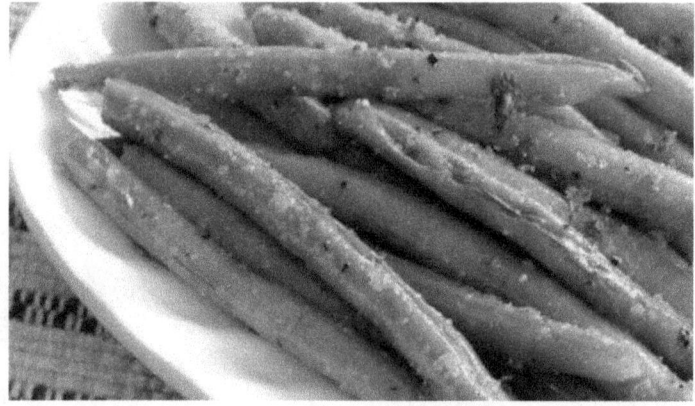

4. Add a small whole-wheat roll and use a teaspoon of soft tub margarine.

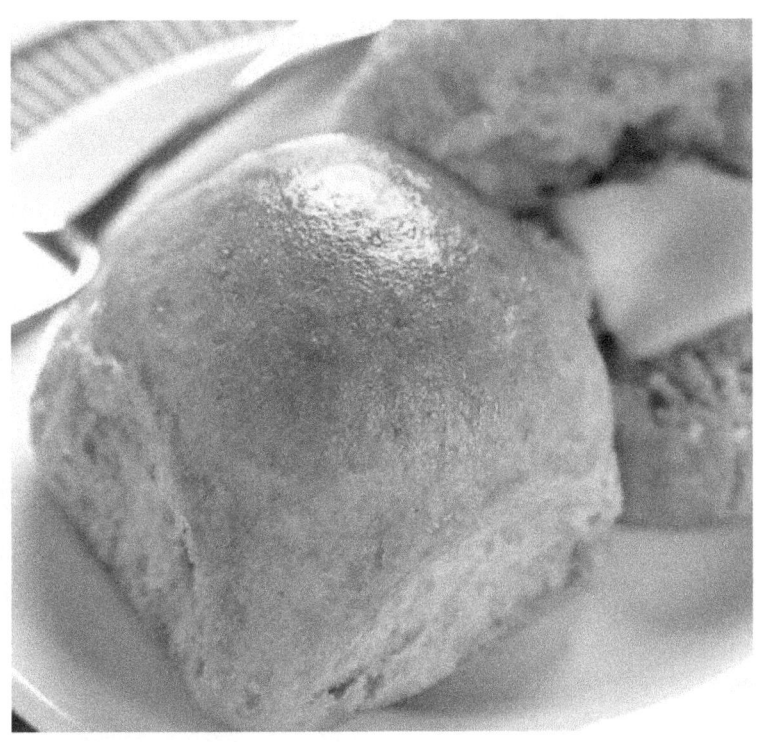

5. Complete your meal with a small apple.

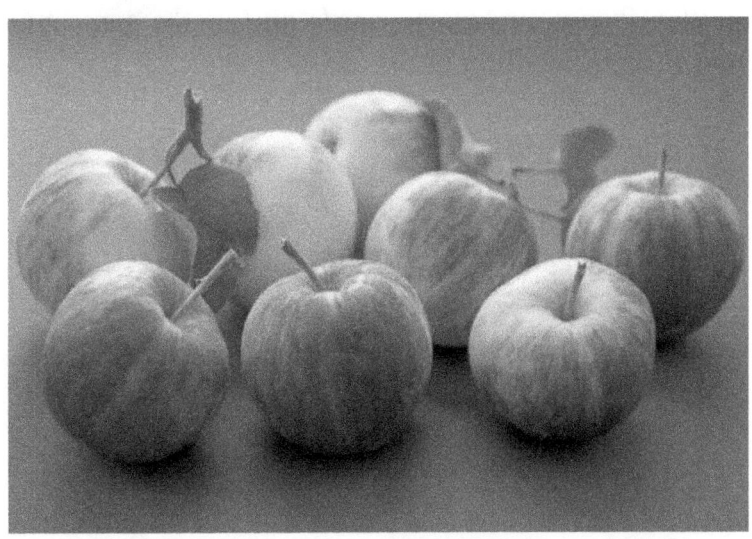

6. For the liquid intake, drink a cup of low-fat milk.

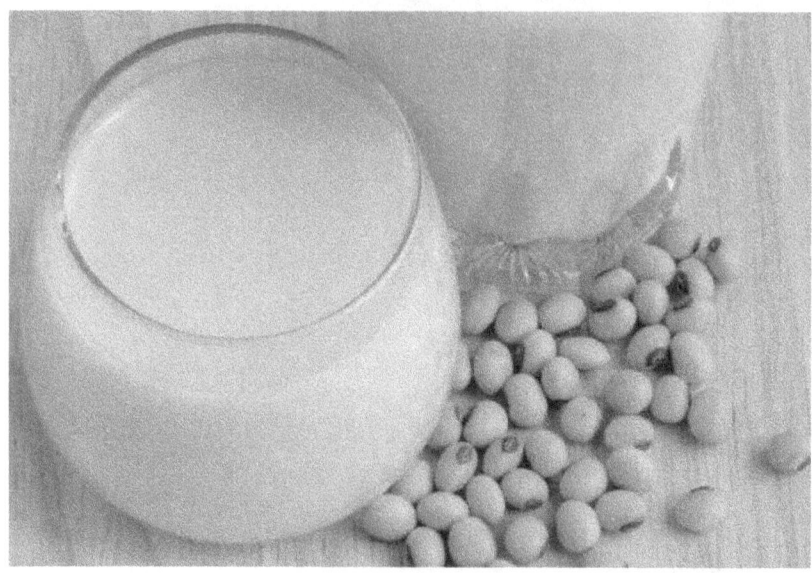

Tip

The total sodium intake for these whole dinners is ~578 mg. This will suffice your calorie needs and at the same time, it will maintain the sodium levels too.

Meal Plan

Day 2

For day 2 of the week, following is the meal plan you need to adhere to.

Breakfast

To begin your day, you need the right kind of meal plans. Here is what you can eat to make the most of your day.

1. A whole-wheat bagel, preferably mini. You can have it along with a tablespoon of peanut butter for extra delicious taste.

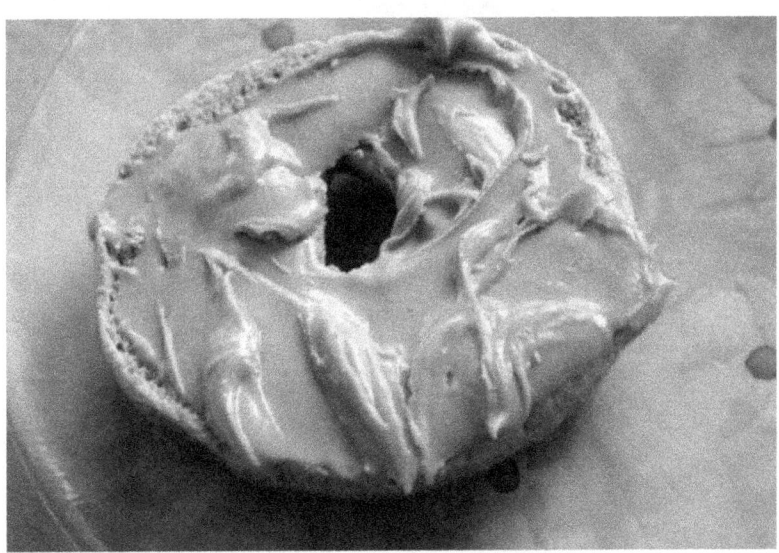

2. ½ cup of instant oatmeal as it is rich in energy.

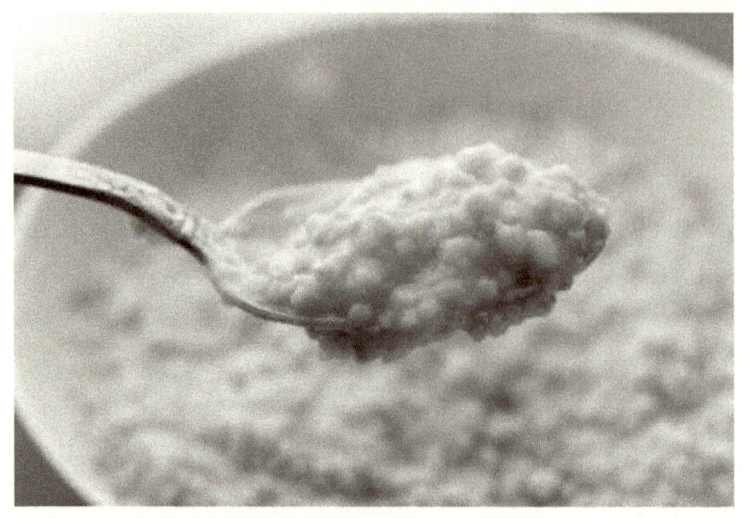

3. 1 cup of low-fat milk

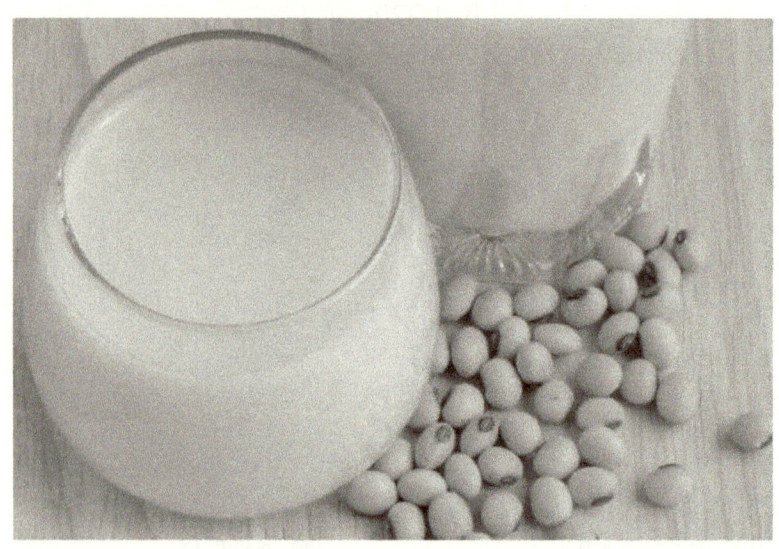

4. 1 medium sized banana

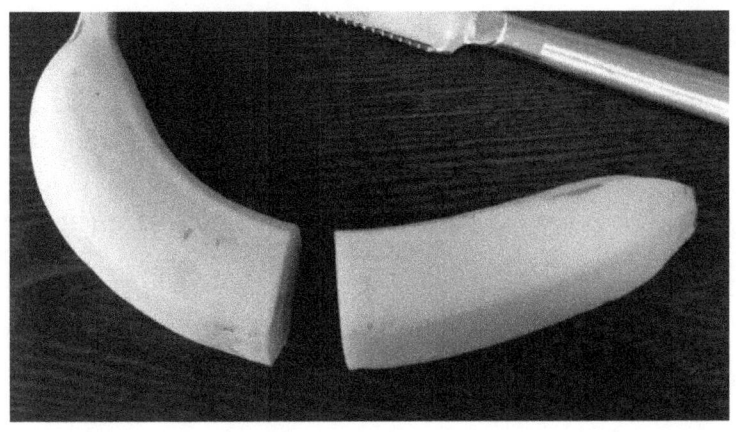

Tip

The overall sodium intake of this whole meal measures 327 mg.

Lunch

For your lunch, you can have a chicken sandwich.

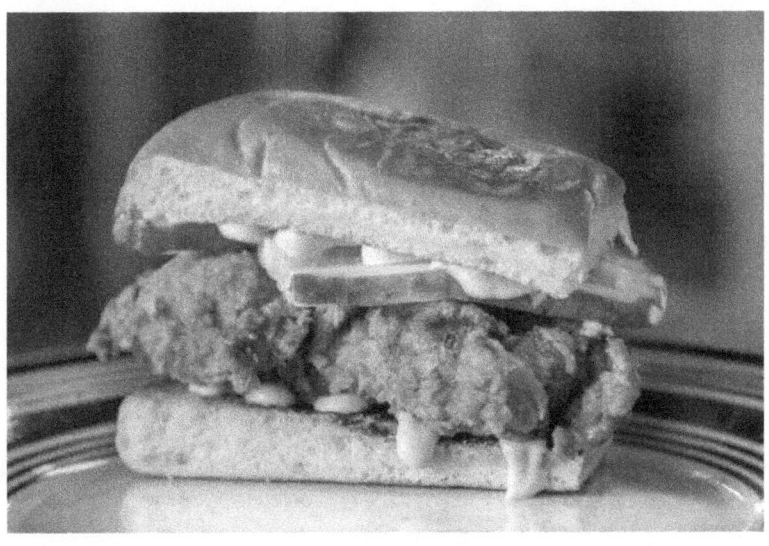

Ingredients

- 4 pounds of cut up whole chicken, 2 pieces
- ¾ cup of prepared mustard
- 5 tablespoons of brown sugar and minced garlic each
- 5 tablespoons of honey
- 12 hamburger buns
- 3 tablespoons of liquid smoke flavoring
- ¼ cup of steak sauce
- 1 ½ cups of ketchup
- 4 tablespoons of lemon juice
- Salt and pepper as per need.

Instructions

1. Take a large pot and place chicken in it. Make sure to bring the pot to boil and cook it thoroughly until the chicken can come off the bone easily.

2. Take a saucepan and place it over medium heat. Make sure to mix the ketchup, brown sugar, garlic, mustard, and steak sauce, and honey, liquid smoke and lemon juice.

3. Season the mixture with salt and pepper. Bring the mixture to gentle boil and let it simmer for around 10 minutes. Keep it aside so that you let the flavors to blend thoroughly.

4. After the chicken has been done, remove all the meat from bones and then chop them into small pieces.

5. Take a plan and add sauce to it. Cook it for nearly 15 minutes as this will allow the sauce to thoroughly soak into the chicken. Pour the barbecued chicken into buns and serve.

To supplement the chicken dish, you can have a cup of cantaloupe and a cup of apple juice. This will add the fruit intake to your diet and make your lunch complete.

Dinner

For dinner, we will have a combination of fruits salad and other stuff. Here is a list of things you need to have.

1. ½ cup of canned pears, preferably a juice pack.

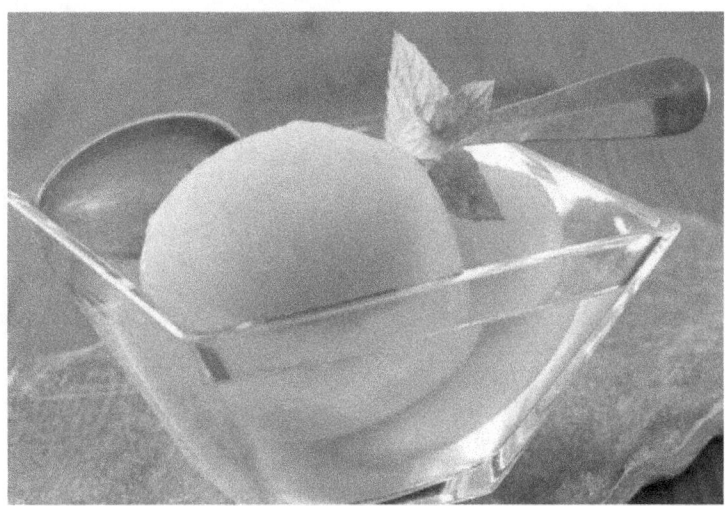

2. ½ cup of corn which was stored frozen and was later thoroughly cooked.

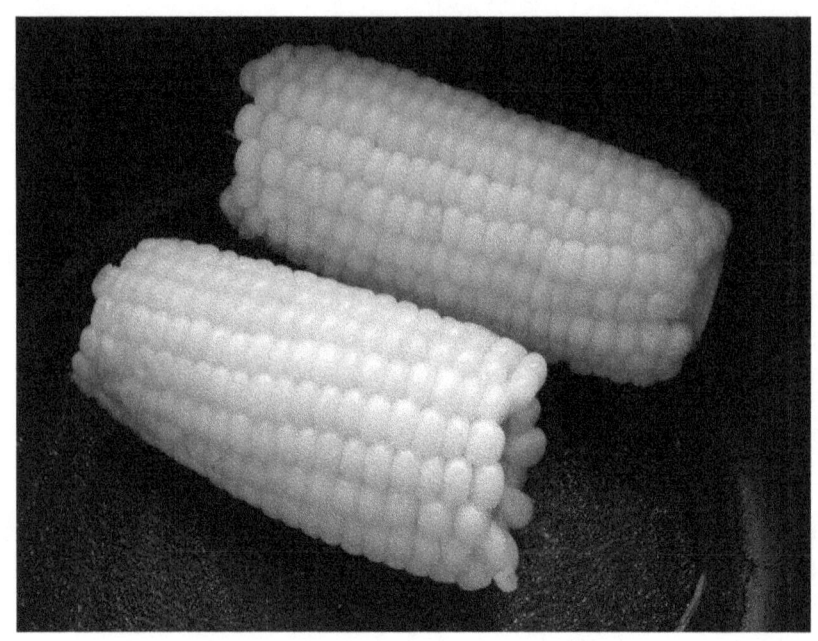

3. Spinach salad

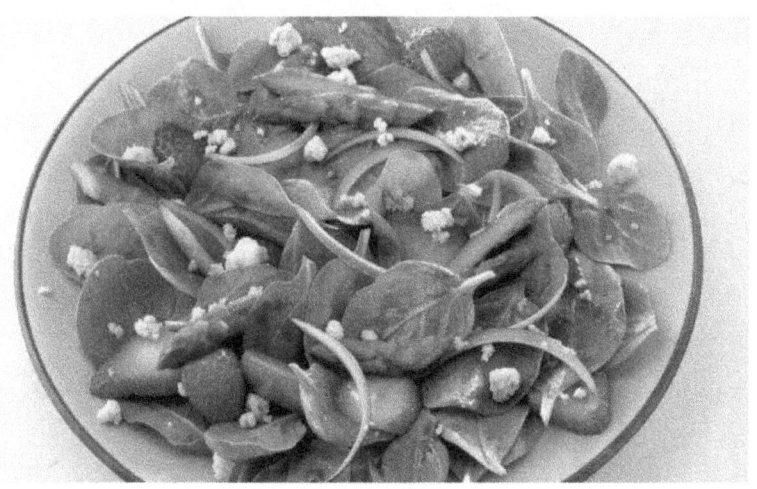

4. 1 cup of spaghetti

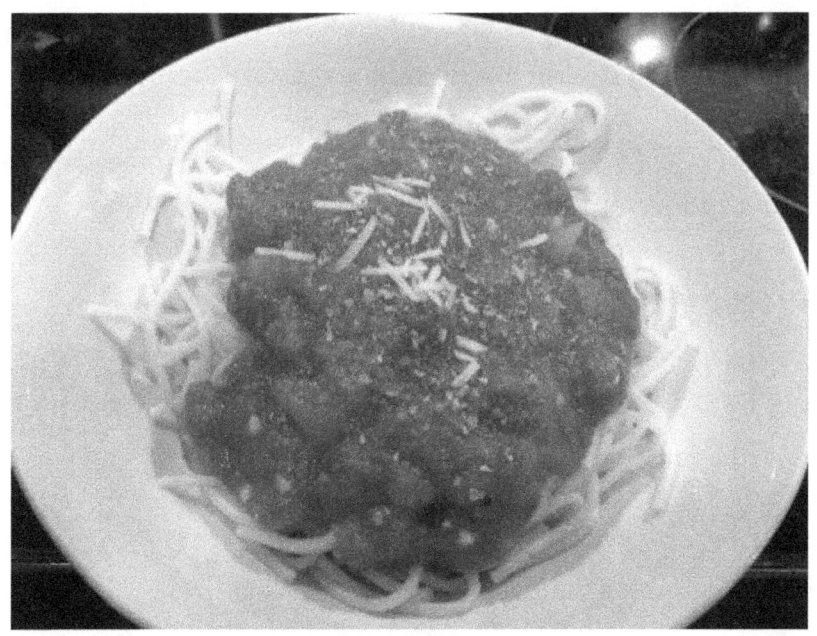

In order to make spinach salad, you will need the following.

Ingredients

- 1 cup of fresh spinach leaves.
- ¼ cup of freshly grated carrots.
- ¼ cup of sliced mushrooms which are fresh.
- 1 tablespoon of vinaigrette salad dressing.

Instructions

1. Take a clean bowl and mix all these ingredients in it except for salad dressing. Make sure that the spinach leaves, carrots and mushrooms have been finely chopped and diced.

2. When you have thoroughly mixed the ingredients, pour the salad dressing at the top. Serve.

For the cup of spaghetti, you will need ¾ cup of vegetarian spaghetti sauce and the recipe for the same is as follows.

Vegetarian Spaghetti Sauce

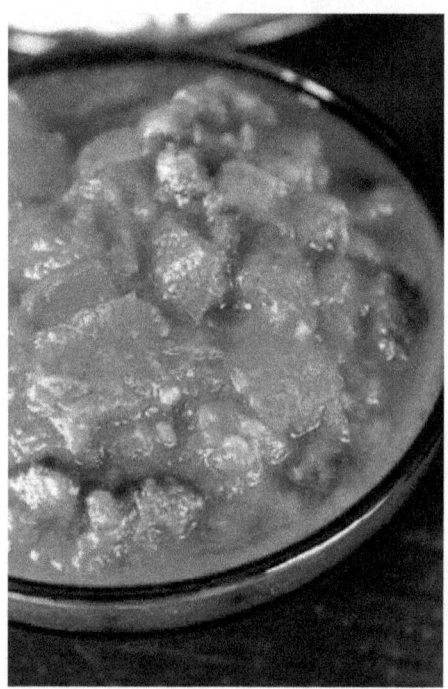

Ingredients

- 2 small chopped onions
- 2 medium sized tomato which have been chopped
- 1 ¼ cup of sliced zucchini
- 1 tablespoon of dried basil and dried oregano
- 1 can of tomato sauce weighing 8 oz

- 1 can of tomato paste weighing 6 oz
- 2 tablespoon of olive oil
- 3 chopped garlic cloves
- 1 cup of water

Instructions

1. Take a medium sized skillet and heat oil in it. Now, sauté onions, zucchini and garlic in the oil for 5 minutes while keeping it on medium heat.

2. Add all the remaining ingredients and simmer it for 45 minutes keeping it covered. Serve over spaghetti.

Tip

In order to cut down the sodium intake, you can use a 6 oz can of tomato paste which comes salt free.

I hope that you are enjoying this book so far, and if you could spare 30 seconds, I would greatly appreciate you leaving a review on Amazon.com.

Meal Plan

Day 3

On the third day of the week, you can adhere to the following to ensure that your diet plan for regulating blood pressure stays intact.

Breakfast

The breakfast for day 3 can be same as that of day 1 because there is no harm in repeating meals alternately. Following are the things you can eat for your breakfast and kick start your day in the right manner.

1. 3/4th cup of bran flakes cereal. Make it a point to use a medium sized banana along with a cup of low-fat milk with it. This makes a good breakfast and will fill your empty stomach without substantially adding calories and sodium to your diet.

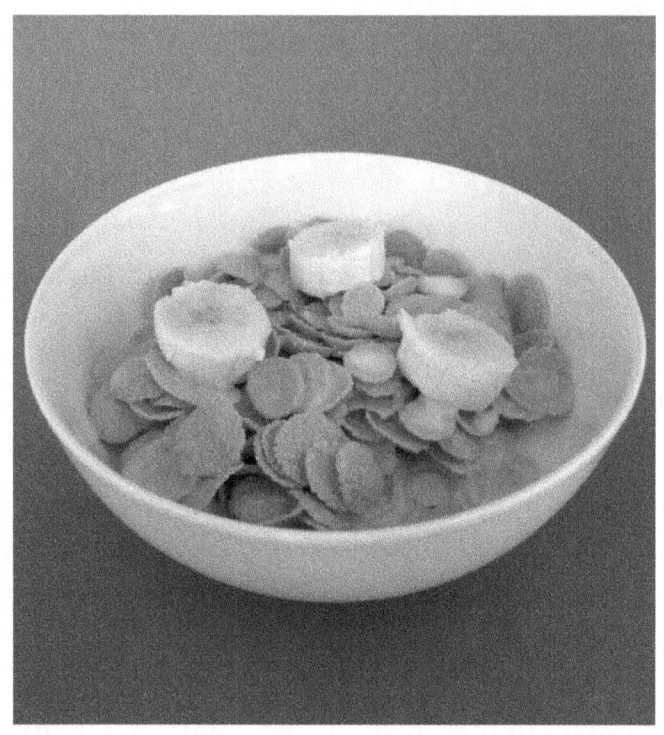

2. To fill the stomach further, you can have a slice of whole wheat bread and make sure to add a teaspoon of soft tub margarine to it.

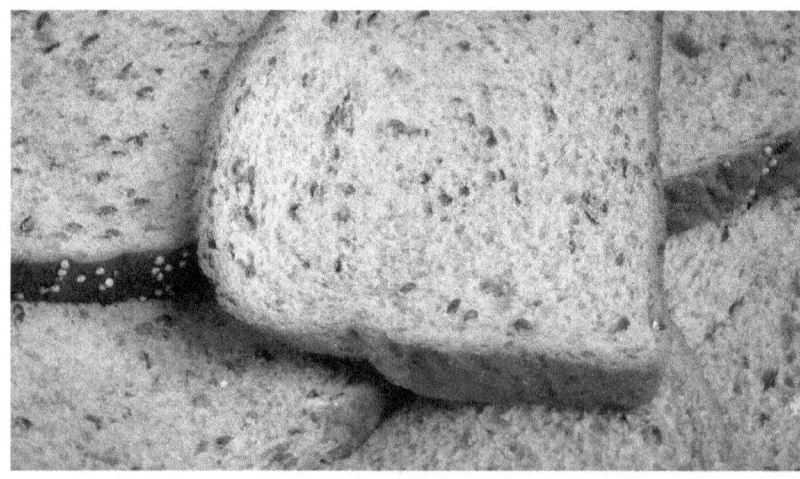

3. As far as liquid intake is concerned, wash your meal with a cup of nutritious orange juice.

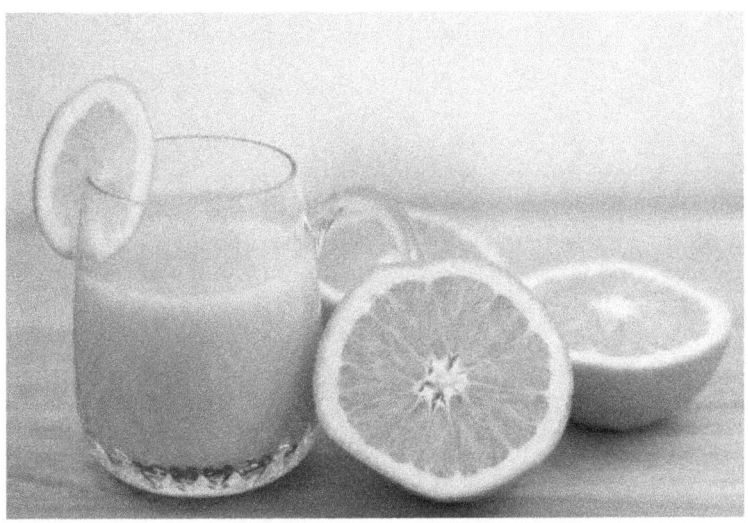

This meal is so planned that you will be able to get a blend of grains, dairy products, fruits and even necessary fats and oil as well.

Lunch

For your lunch, you can have a combination of sandwich and salad. Here are the meals you can have to satiate your food buds.

1. Beef barbecue sandwich.
2. A cup of new potato salad.
3. A medium sized orange; ether raw or in juice form.

Here are the details of how to make the perfect beef barbecue sandwich.

Beef Barbecue Sandwich

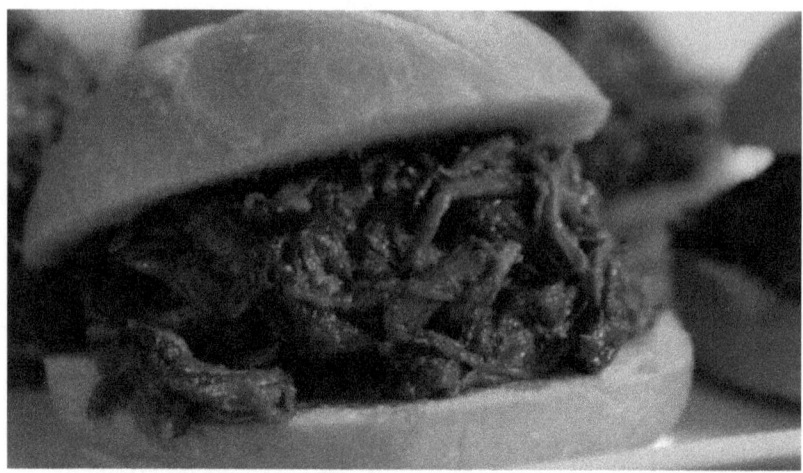

Ingredients

- A boneless roast of beef chuck, weighing nearly 3 pounds.
- 2 tablespoons of Worcestershire sauce.
- 2 tablespoons of Dijon mustard.
- ¼ cup of packed brown sugar.
- ¼ cup of barbecue sauce.
- 1 to 1 ½ cups of ketchup.
- ¼ teaspoon of garlic powder.
- 12 split sandwich buns.
- Sliced onions.
- ½ teaspoon of salt.
- ¼ teaspoon pepper.

Instructions

1. Cut the beef roast into halves and place them in a slow cooker. Take a small bowl and mix ketchup, barbecue sauce, mustard, brown sugar and then the seasonings as well. Pour this mixture over beef.

2. Cover the whole mixture and cook on low for 8 to 10 hours until you find that the meat has become tender. Now, remove the meat and let it cool.

3. Shred the beef and return it to the slow cooker. Cover the same and let it cook or 15 minutes. Place ½ cup of the mixture on each bun and serve it with sliced onions.

If you are wondering how to make the best potato salad, here is the recipe you can use.

Potato Salad

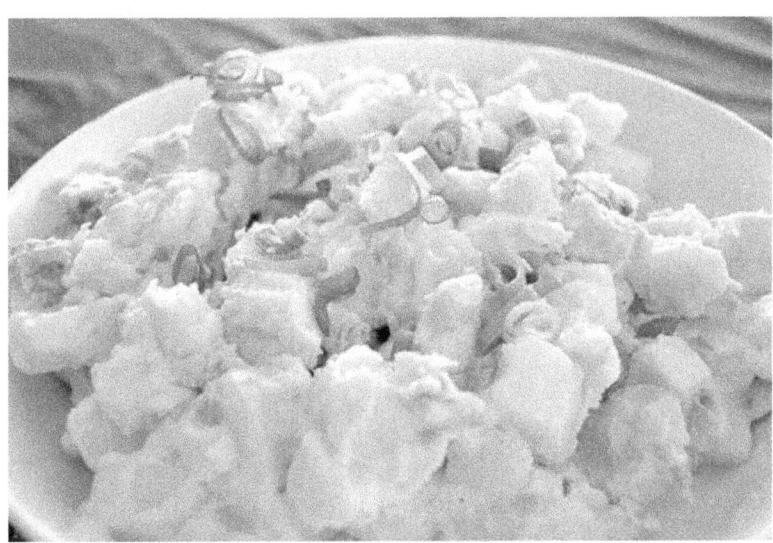

Ingredients

- 5 cups of new potatoes preferably small in size.
- ¼ teaspoon of black pepper.
- 2 tablespoon of olive oil.
- ¼ cup of chopped green onions.
- 1 teaspoon of dried dill weed.

Instructions

1. Clean the potatoes thoroughly. Boil them for nearly 20 minutes until they become tender. Drain and cool the potatoes for nearly 20 minutes.

2. Cut the potatoes and mix it thoroughly with onions, spices and olive oil. Refrigerate it and serve when needed.

These meals make the perfect lunch and will satiate your calorie needs as well.

Dinner

In order to have a complete meal during dinner, you can have the following.

1. 3 oz of cod. Cod makes an excellent meal as it will fill your stomach and at the same time is a healthy choice too. Make sure to add a teaspoon of lemon juice for the extra taste.

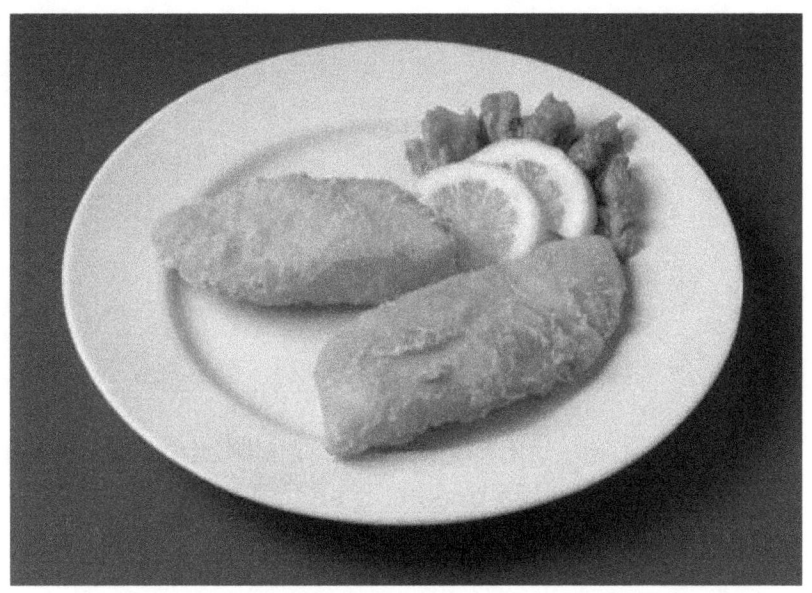

2. You can always team it with ½ cup of brown rice.

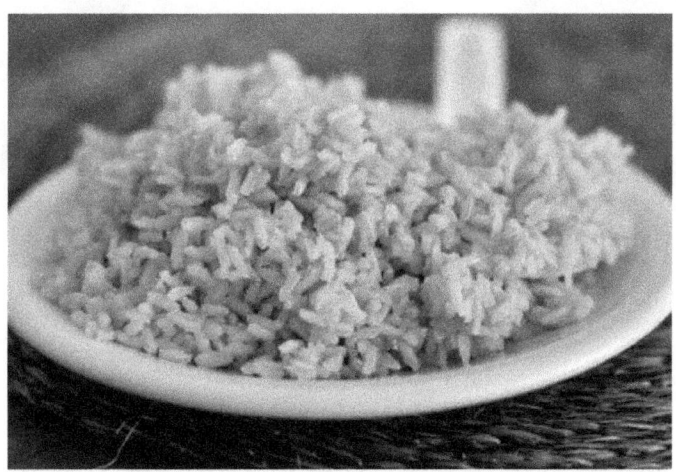

3. A cup of spinach which was earlier frozen and has been cooked thoroughly. It should be sautéed with a teaspoon of canola oil and you can add a tablespoon of silvered almond as well.

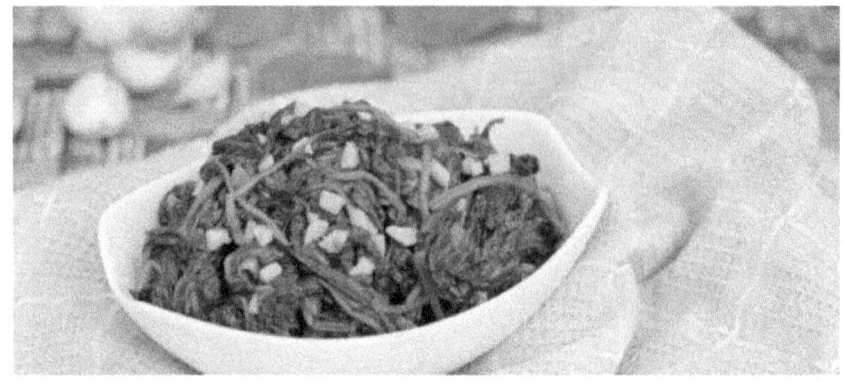

4. To top it all, you can have a small cornbread muffin. You can use oil in making it and add a teaspoon of soft tub margarine.

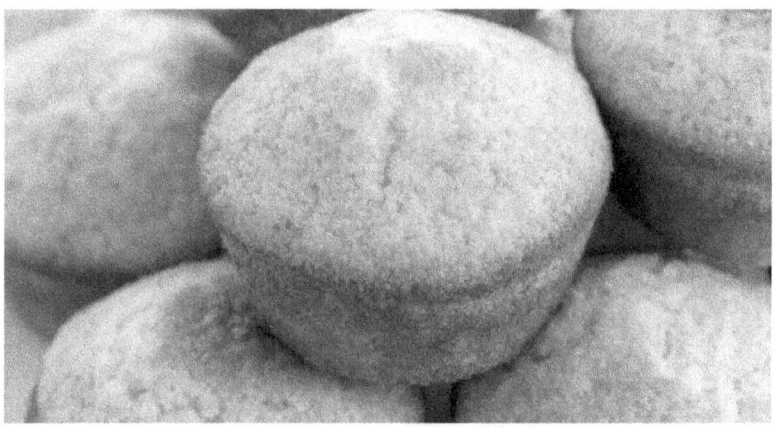

Tip

This complete meal comprises of just 405 mg of sodium and will thus keep your blood pressure levels in check.

Meal Plan

Day 4

Welcome to Day 4 of your 7-day meal plan. You have managed to control the sodium levels so far by sticking to the diet chart for the first three days. It is easier to follow the meal plans now as your body starts getting habituated to the same.

Breakfast

For your breakfast, you can have the following combination of meals.

1. A slice of whole wheat bread. You can use a teaspoon of soft tub margarine to go along with it.

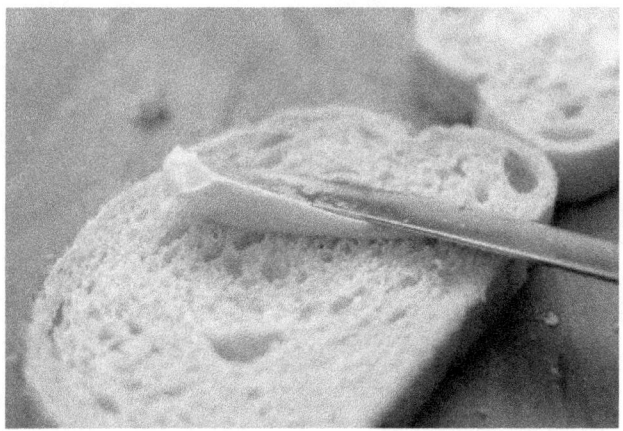

2. 1 cup of fat free fruit yogurt. Make sure that it contains no added sugar.

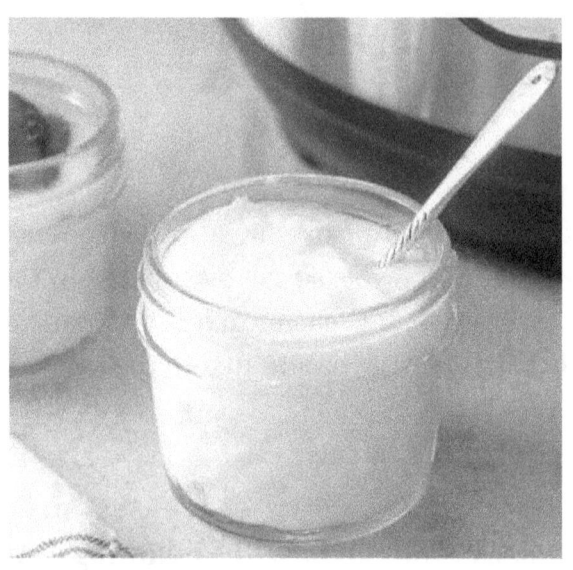

3. 1 medium sized peach.

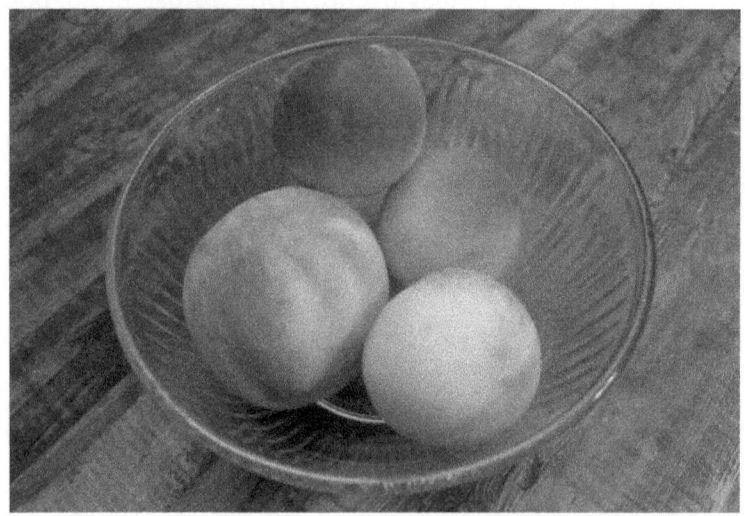

4. ½ cup of grape juice. This is important because having fruits in the morning gives your body the much-needed energy.

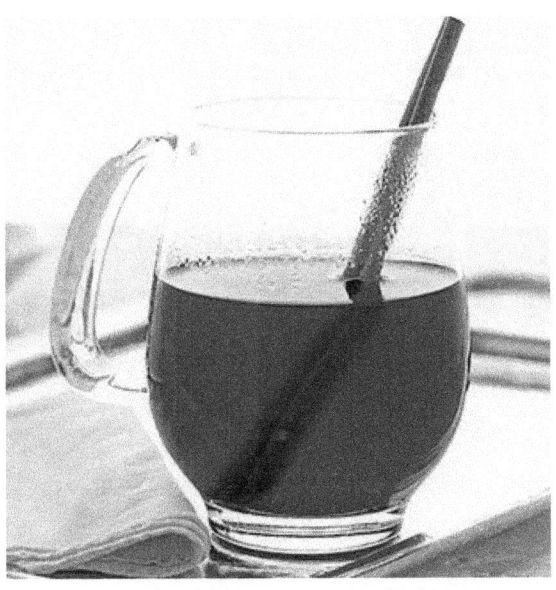

Lunch

For your lunch meal, you can have a combination of the following.

1. Ham and cheese sandwich.

2. 1 carrot stick

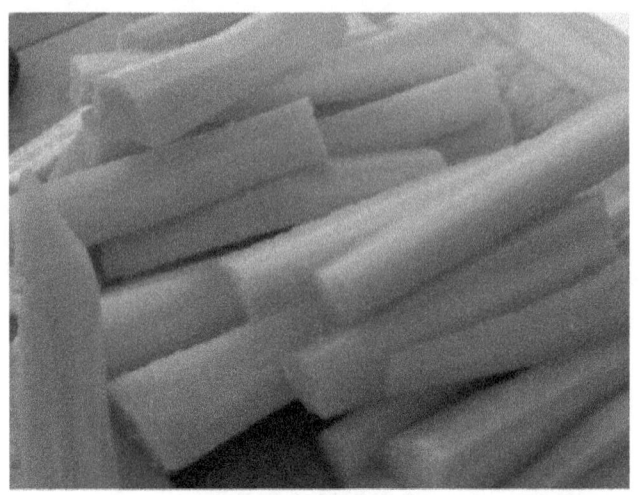

Those who do not know how to prepare the best ham and cheese sandwich can get hold of the recipe here.

Ham and Cheese Sandwich

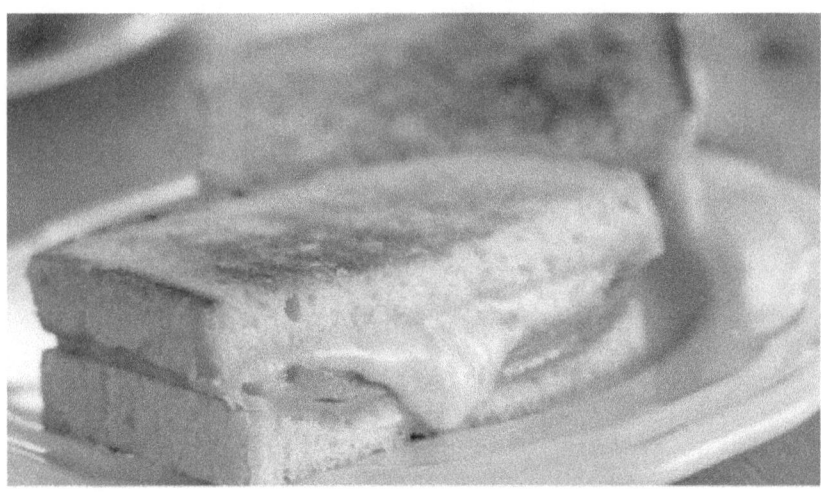

Ingredients

- 50 gm of softened butter.

- 100 gm of thinly sliced ham.
- 4 thick slice of white bread.
- Dressed salad leaves for the purpose of serving.
- 80 gm of thinly sliced cheese.
- 2 teaspoons of Dijon mustard

Instructions

1. Place 2 slices of bread on a board. Take a small bowl and add mustard and 20 g of butter in it. Mix it through. Spread this paste over bread. Top the whole mix with ham and cheese. Season it with the use of salt and pepper.

2. Spread the leftover bread with mustard, sandwich and butter together and press it together. Take a non-stick frying pan and pour 15 gm butter in it. Heat the pan over medium heat.

3. Place 1 of the sandwiches in a pan and cook for a couple of minutes until it turns golden. Repeat the same with the other sandwich and the leftover butter. Serve the sandwich with salad.

Dinner

For your dinner, rice seems to be a great choice. We are going to list down the details of the things you can have to keep the blood pressure in check.

1. Chicken and Spanish rice.

2. A cup of cantaloupe chunks.

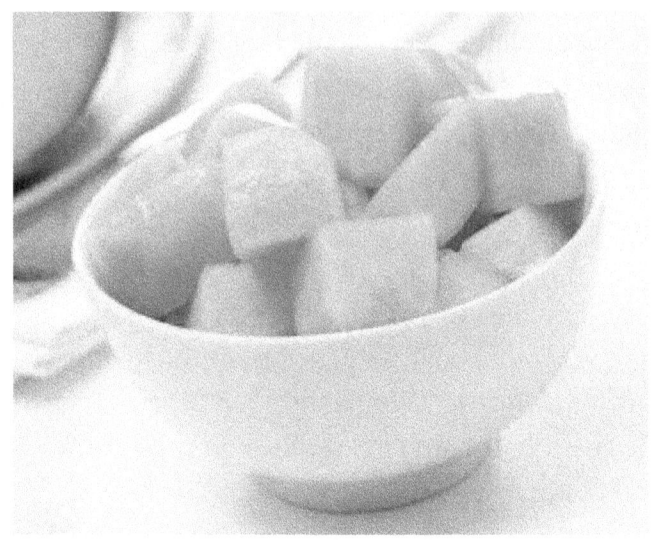

3. A cup of low-fat milk

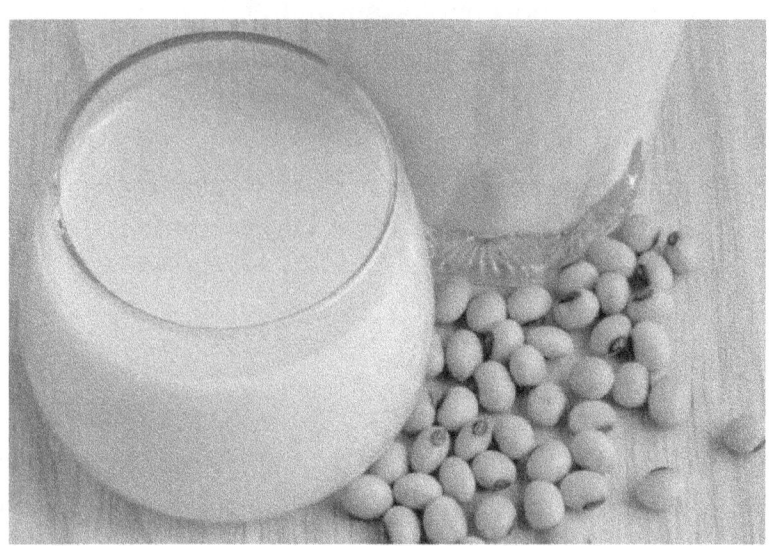

If you are looking for the right recipe that can help you cook delicious chicken and Spanish rice, here is the perfect recipe for you.

Chicken and Spanish Rice

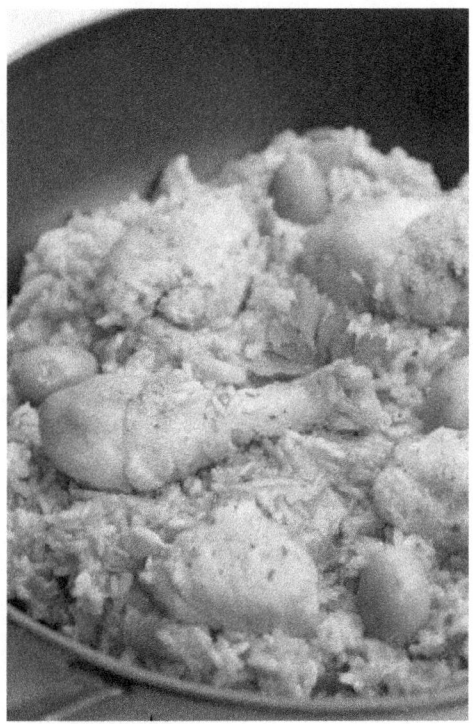

Ingredients

- A cup of chopped onions.
- 5 cups of brown rice which has been cooked in unsalted water.
- ¼th cup of green peppers.
- 3 ½ cups of chicken breast which has been thoroughly cooked and has the skin and bone removed as well.

- 1 can of tomato sauce weighing 8 oz.
- 1 1/4th teaspoon of minced garlic.
- 2 teaspoons of vegetable oil.
- 1 teaspoon of chopped parsley.
- ½ teaspoon of black pepper

Instructions

1. Take a large skillet and sauté onion and green peppers in oil for 5 minutes over medium heat.

2. Add tomato sauce along with spices and heat it thoroughly. Now add cooked rice and chicken and heat again. Serve

Tip

You can cut down on the sodium by using a 4 oz can of salt free tomato sauce and another can of regular tomato sauce.

Enjoying this book?

Check out my other best sellers!

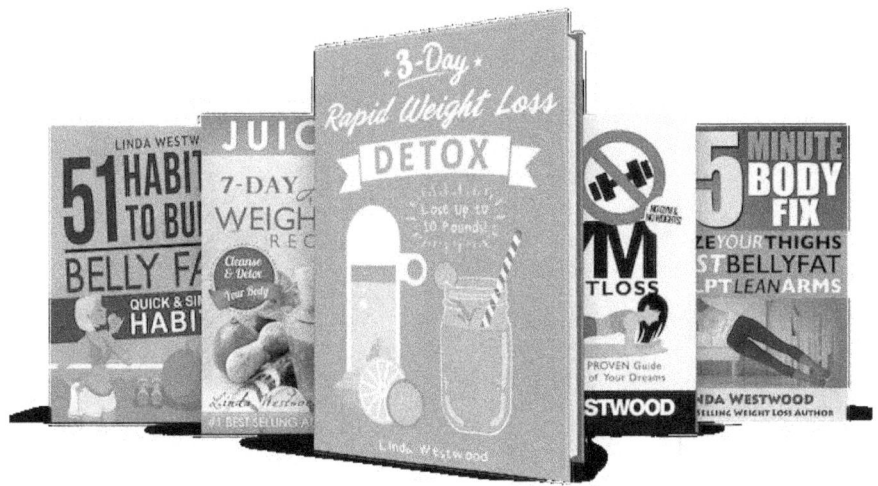

Get your next book on sale here:

TopFitnessAdvice.com/go/books

Meal Plan

Day 5

When you have reached day 5, you have made quite a lot of progress in the DASH meal plan. So, keep on following the same.

Breakfast

For your breakfast, you can have the following meals.

1. A cup of whole oats rings cereal. You should team it with a medium sized banana and a cup of low-fat milk.

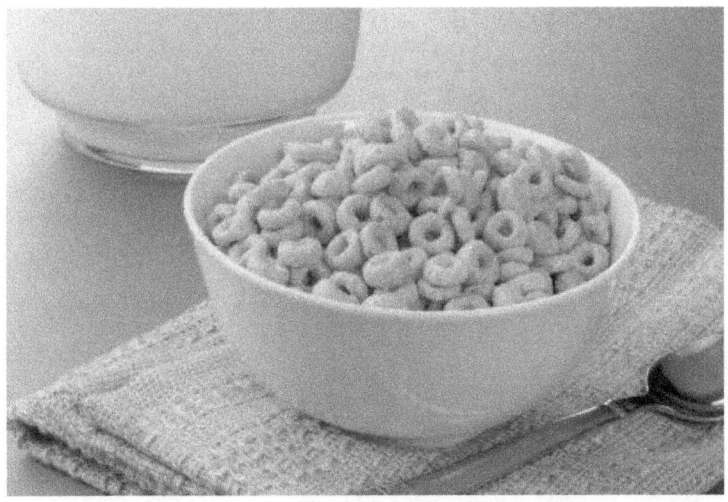

2. A medium sized raisin bagel. Add a tablespoon of peanut butter.

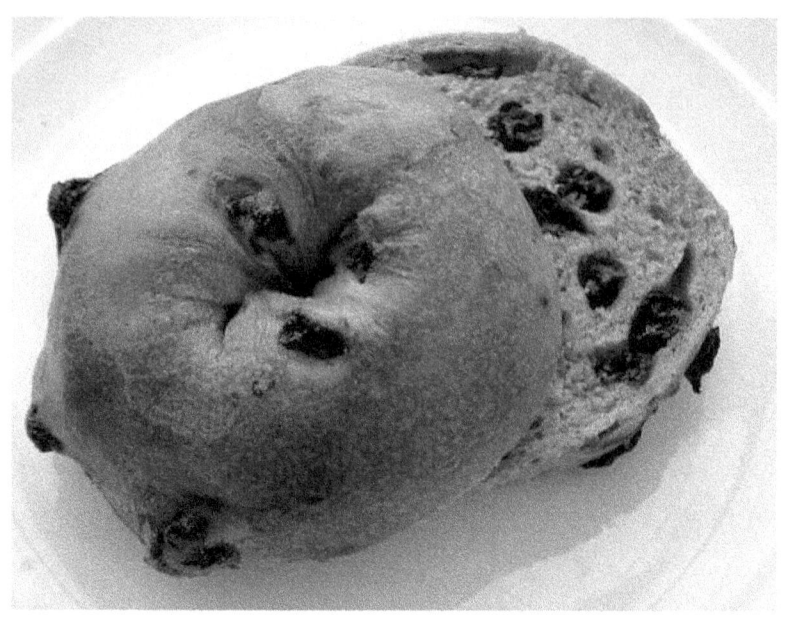

3. A cup of orange juice to wash off the meal.

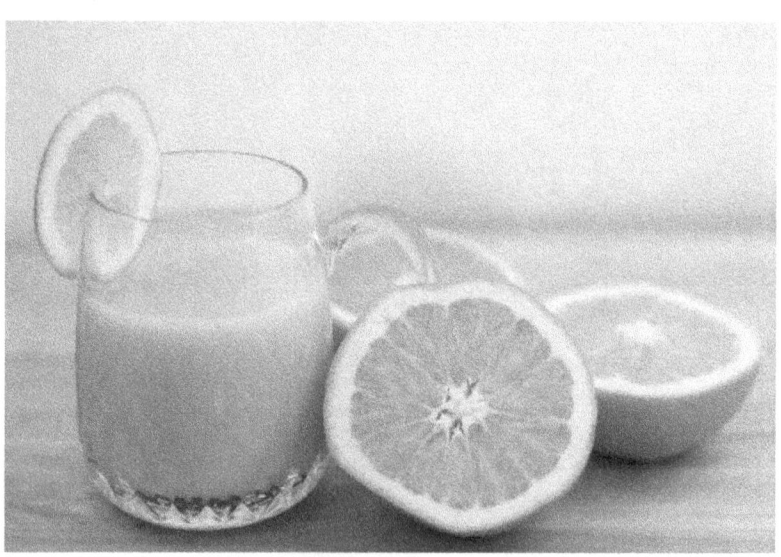

Tip

The total sodium intake for this meal is 739 mg. This diet is pretty balanced and will ensure that the energy needs of your body will be thoroughly fulfilled.

Lunch

Salad and fruits seem to be one of the best combinations for lunch as it gives you the right potion which will help you in your growth.
Here are the meals you can have.

1. Tuna salad plate.

2. ½ cup of canned pineapple, preferably choose a juice pack.

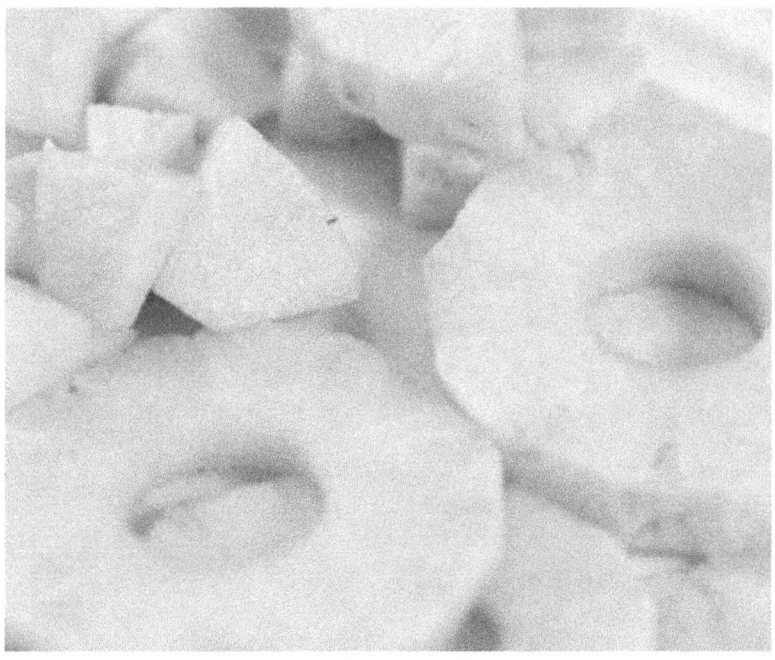

3. 1 tablespoons of almond

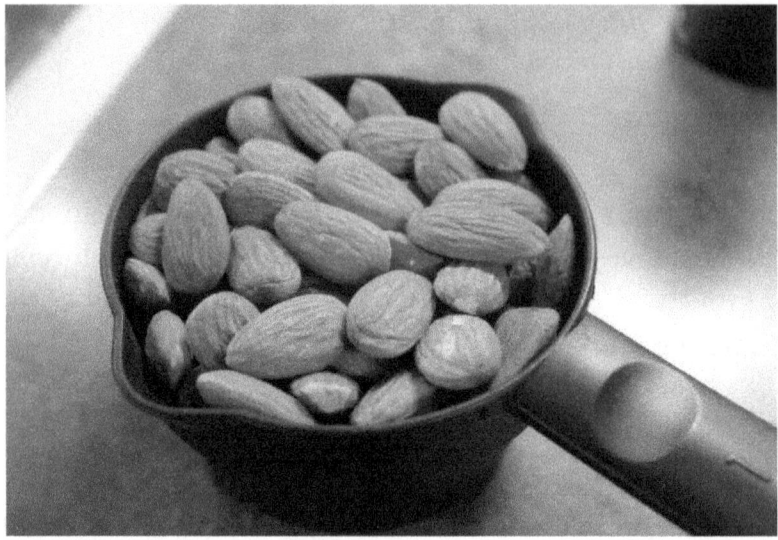

Those who are wondering how to make the best tuna cup salad can go through the following recipe.

Tuna salad

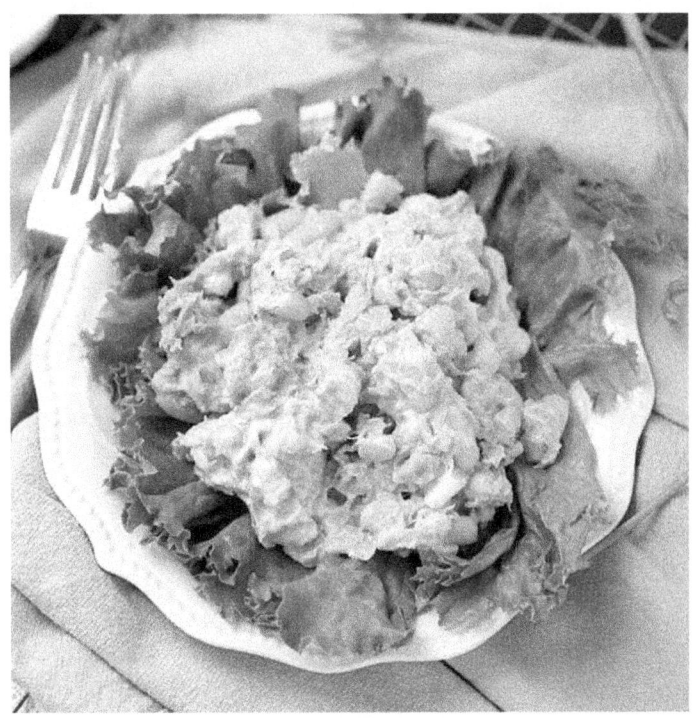

Ingredients

- Two cans of tuna weighing 6 oz, water pack.
- 1/3 cup of chopped green onions.
- ½ cup of finely chopped raw celery.
- 6 1/2 tablespoon of low-fat mayonnaise.

Instructions

1. Take the tuna cans and rinse them for 5 minutes. Break them nicely with help of a fork.

2. Add onion, mayonnaise and celery to it and mix thoroughly. Serve.

This lunch meal should keep you full till dinner and at the same time; it will not impact your sodium consumption levels too.

Dinner

For your dinner, you can let your food buds enjoy the best turkey meatloaf along with other meals too. Here is a list of things you should eat.

1. Turkey meatloaf.

2. A small whole wheat roll.

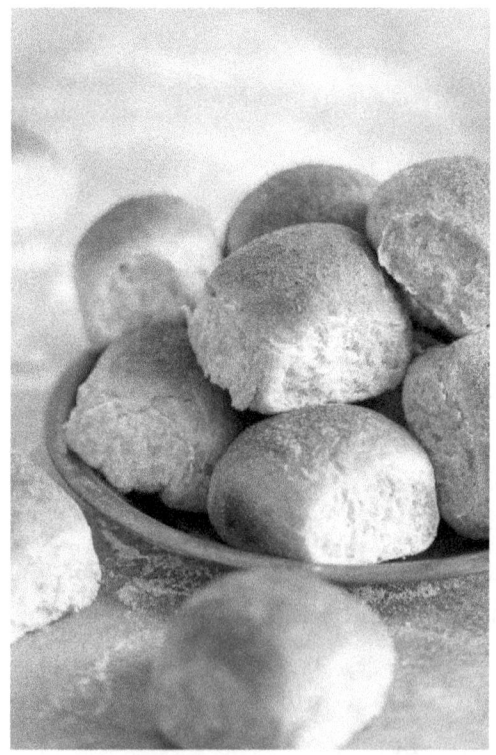

3. 1 cup of collard greens which has been sautéed with the help if 1 teaspoon of canola oil.

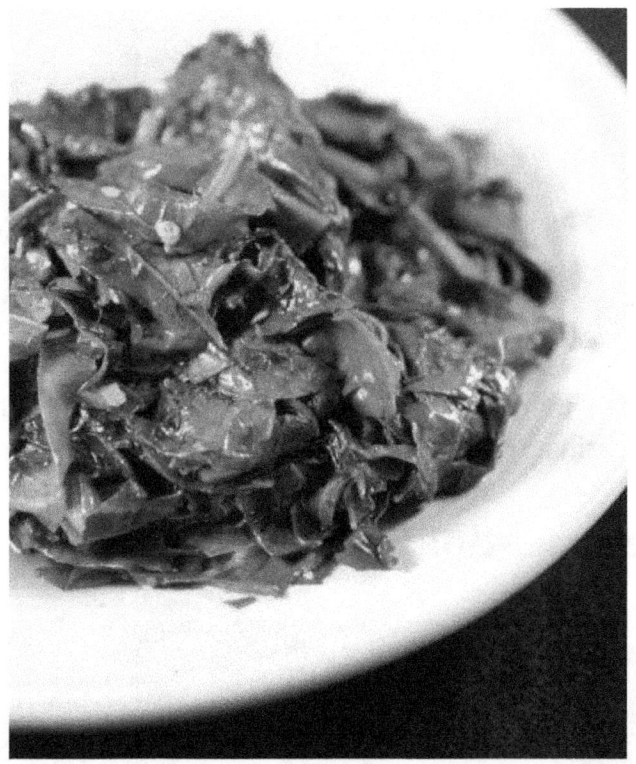

4. A small baked potato. You can add a tablespoon of fat free sour cream along with a tablespoon of cheddar cheese which is natural, grated and has reduced fat levels too.

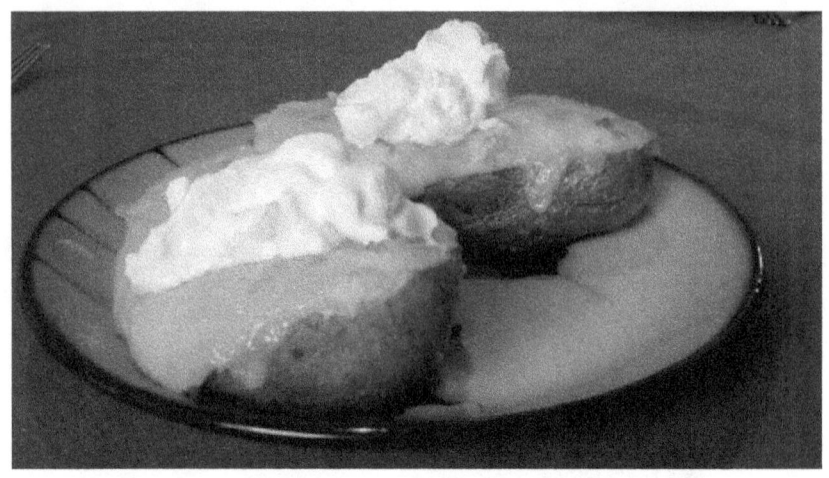

We are now going to talk of ways by which you can make the turkey meatloaf with precision.

Turkey meatloaf

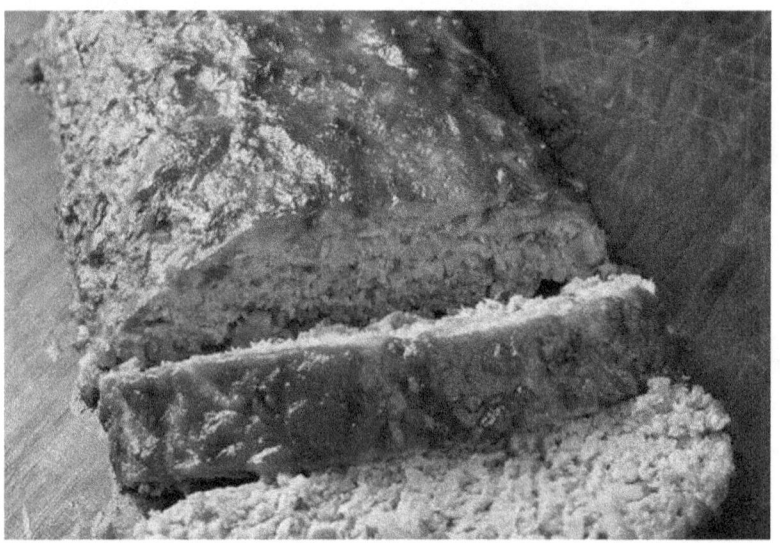

Ingredients

- 1 large egg.
- 1 lb. of lean ground turkey.
- ¼ cup of ketchup.
- 1 tablespoon of dehydrated onion.
- ½ cup of regular dry oats.

Instructions

1. Take all the ingredients in a bowl and mix it well.

2. Take a loaf pan and bake it at 350-degrees Fahrenheit till the loaf is completely baked. Cut it into slices and serve.

Tip

You can further add a cup of fat free fruit yogurt which lacks added sugar, if you want some liquid diet.

Once again, thank you for reading this book, and I hope you're getting a lot of valuable information. I would greatly appreciate it if you could take 30 seconds to leave me a review for this book on Amazon.com.

Meal Plan

Day 6

If you have started the week on a Monday, this would be the weekend meal. You need to make sure that you stick to a disciplined meal even on weekends and do not end up going on an eating spree.

Breakfast

For your weekend breakfast, you can have the following meals.

1. A low-fat granola bar. It is rich in grains and gives your body the much-needed energy.

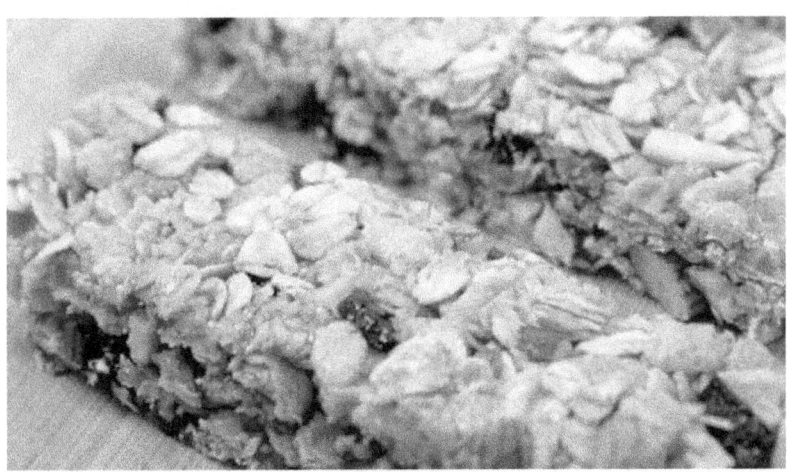

2. 1 medium sized banana

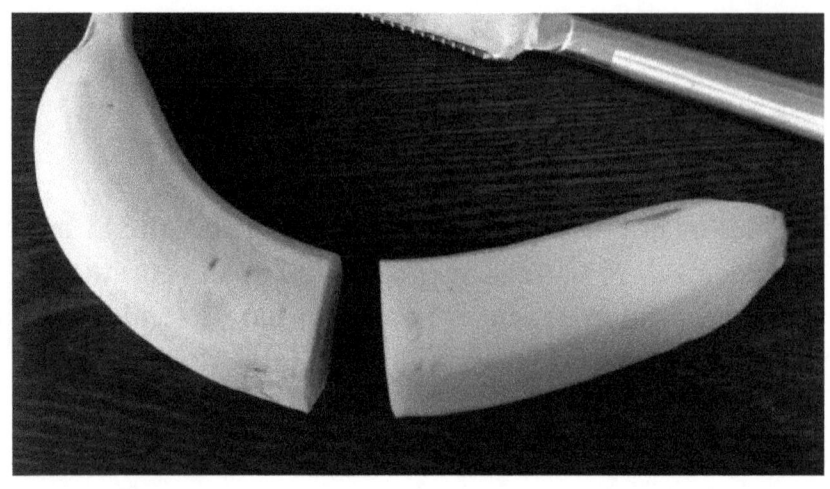

3. ½ cup of fat free fruit yogurt which has no additional sugar in it.

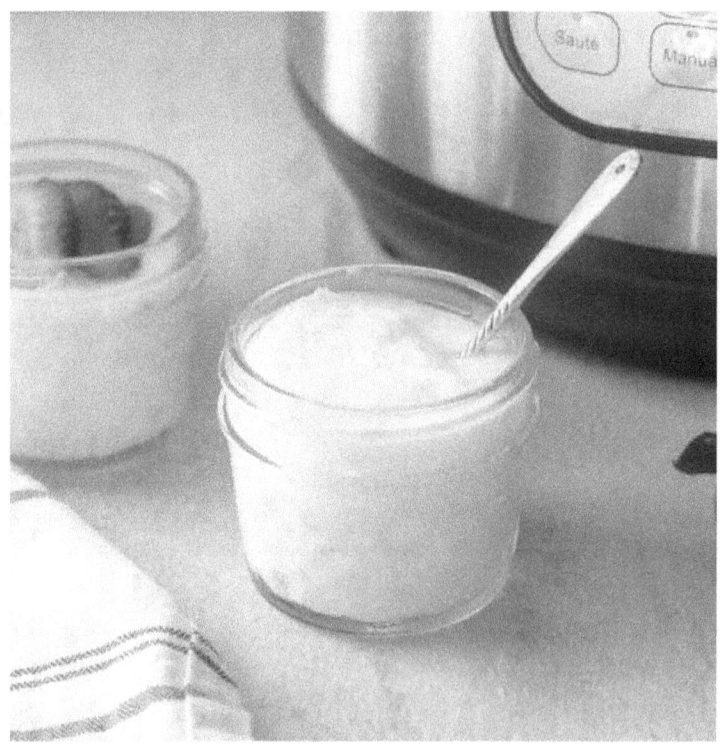

4. A cup of low-fat milk.

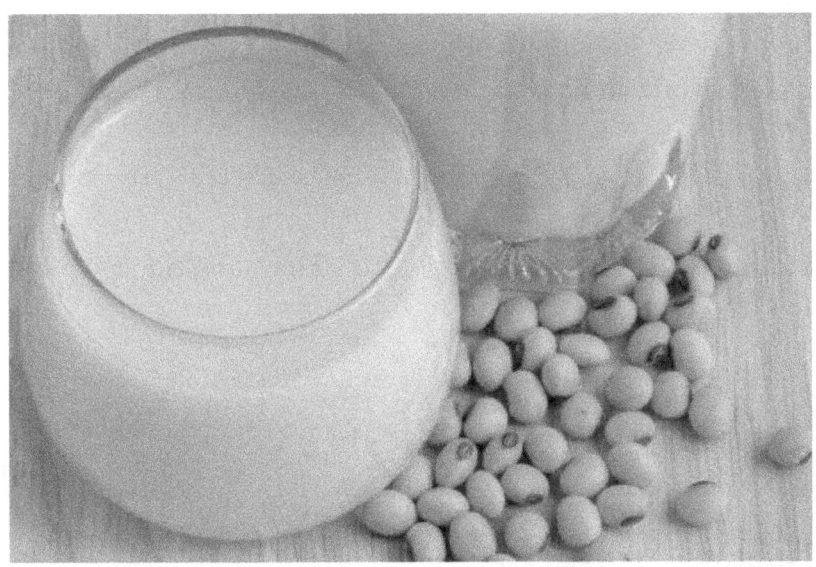

5. A cup of orange juice.

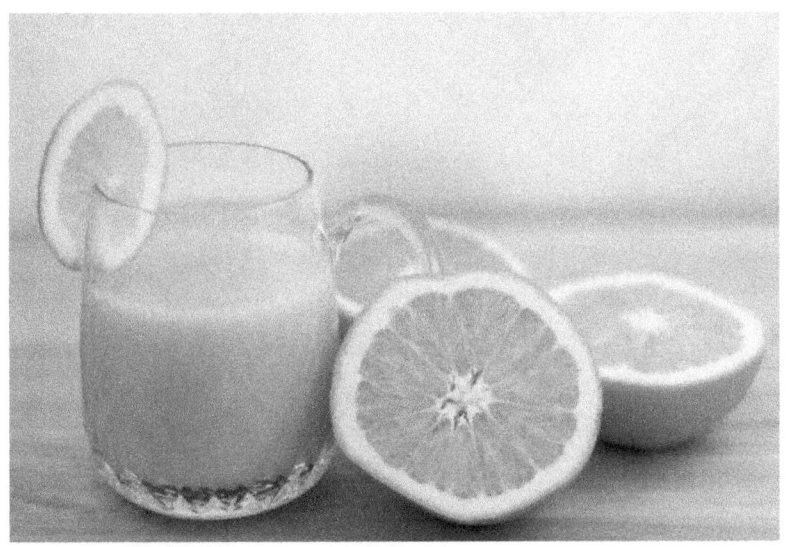

The whole meal comprises of merely 280 mg of sodium.

Lunch

When you are looking for the meals for a lunch, following are the meals you can have.

1. Turkey breast sandwich

2. A cup of steamed broccoli. They should be cooked thoroughly.

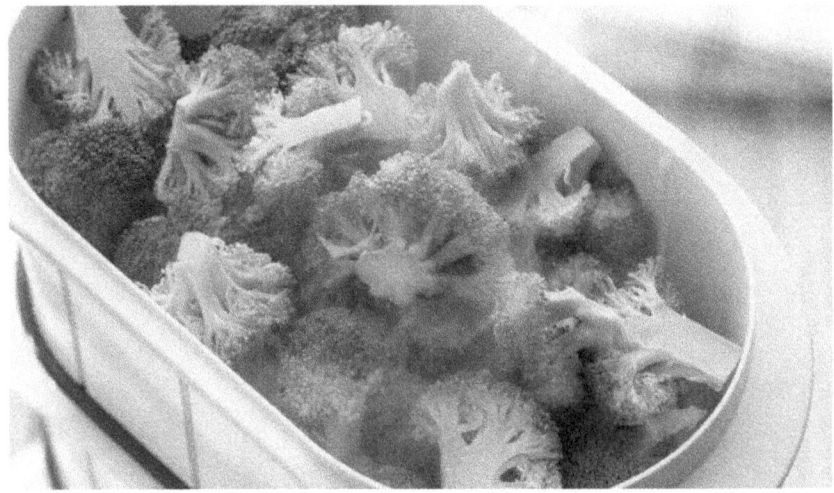

3. A medium sized orange.

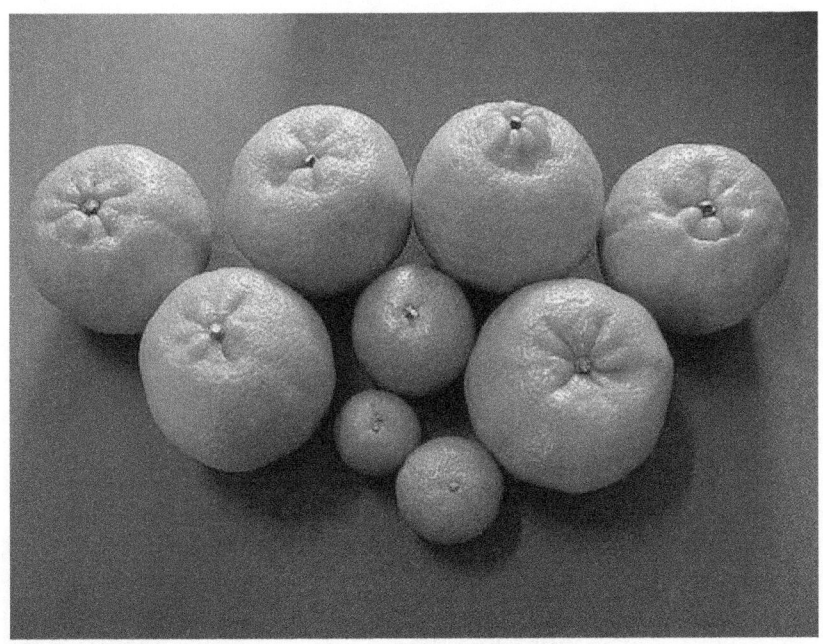

If you want to learn how to make the best turkey breast sandwich, here are the details you need to be acquainted with.

Turkey Breast Sandwich

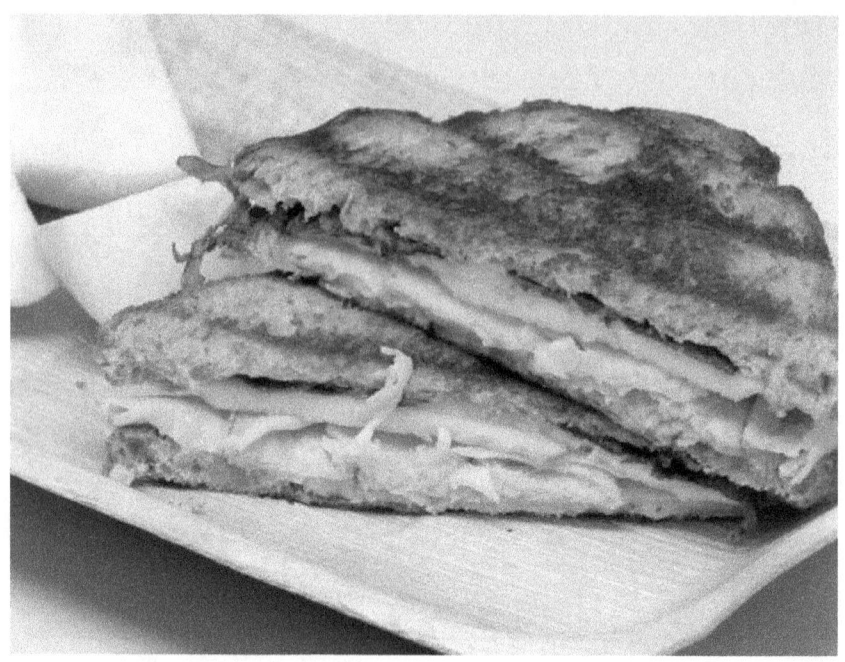

Ingredients

- A sliced loaf of rye bread
- Sliced dill spears
- Pre-sliced turkey breast
- Mayonnaise sauce
- Mustard
- Romaine lettuce
- Black pepper

Instructions

1. Place the bread in a toaster. However, make sure that you do not turn it on. Take the pre-sliced turkey breasts as a platform and place dill spears over it.

2. Add a little black pepper over it. Now, push the toaster down and wait for the toast to be thoroughly cooked.

3. Remove the toast and lift the turkey along with dill and pepper on top and then place it on the toast. Smear both mayonnaise and mustard over it. Flip the bread and then add lettuce to it. Serve

Dinner

If you have a fetish for fish, you are going to love the meal assigned for your dinner.

1. 3 oz of spicy baked fish.

2. A cup of scallion rice.

3. 1 cup of carrots that have been cooked from the frozen state.

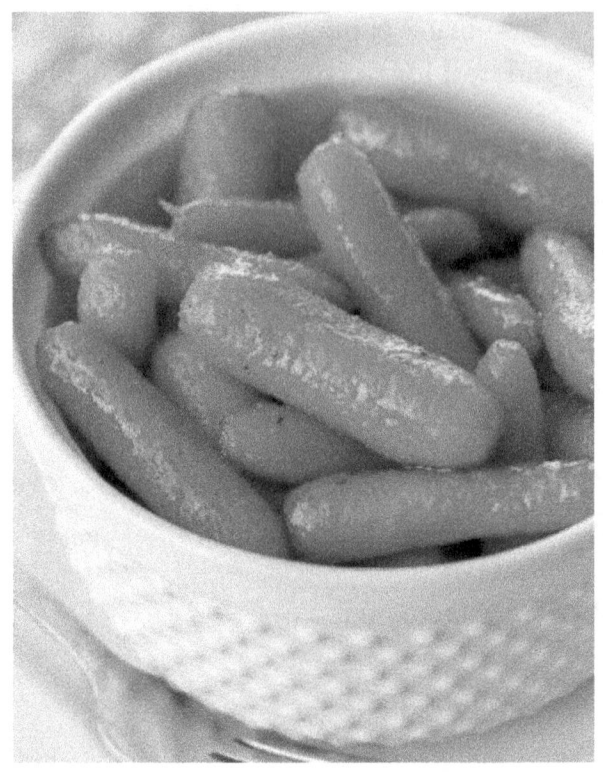

4. A small whole wheat roll which can use a teaspoon of soft tub margarine.

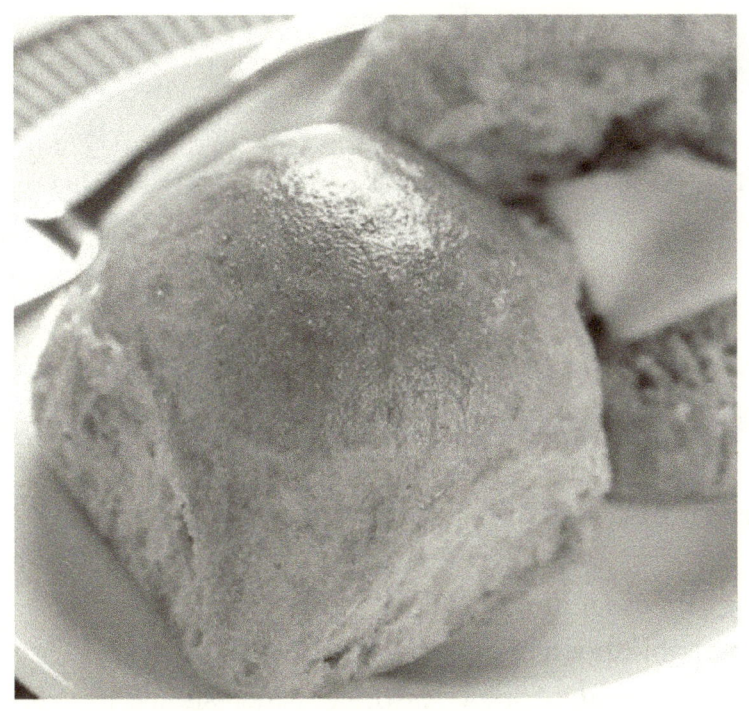

5. As a weekend bonus, you get to have a small cookie.

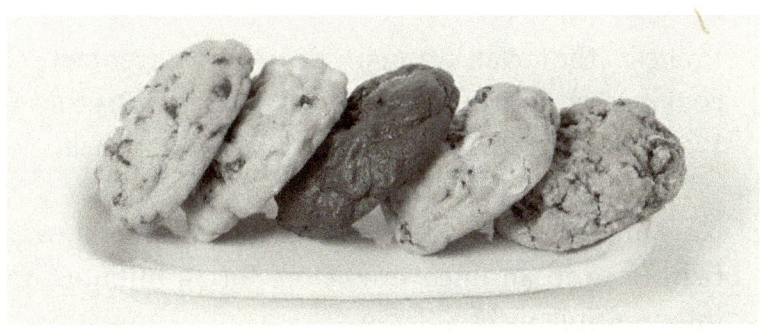

Those who are looking for help to make spicy baked fish can use the following recipe.

Spicy Baked Fish

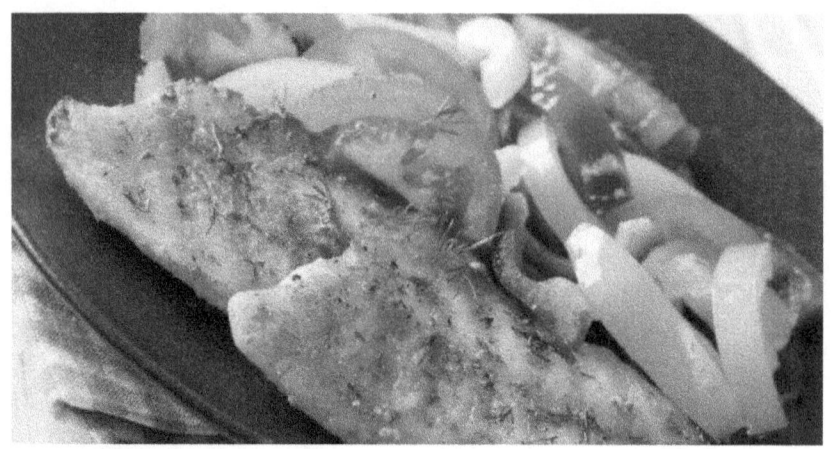

Ingredients

- 1 lb. of salmon fillet.
- 1 tablespoon of olive oil.
- 1 teaspoon of spicy seasoning which should be salt free.

Instructions

1. Preheat the oven to 350 degrees Fahrenheit. Take cooking oil sprays and spray it over a casserole dish. Wash and then dry the fish and place it in a dish.

2. Now mix both oil and seasoning and sprinkle it over the fish. Bake in an uncovered state for 15 minutes. Cut it into multiple pieces. Serve

Tip

Baked fish is best eaten with scallion rice.

If you need a recipe for scallion rice as well, here are the things you need to do.

Scallion Rice

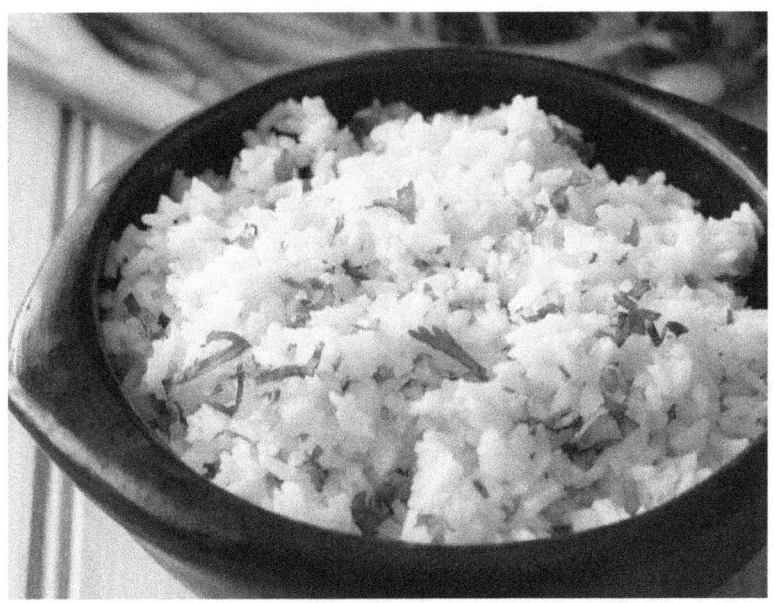

Ingredients

- ¼ cup of chopped scallions.
- 1 ½ teaspoon of bouillon granules which are unsalted.
- 4 ½ cups of rice which have been cooked in unsalted water.

Instructions

1. Cook rice by following the directions which will be listed on the package.

2. Combine all the ingredients and make sure to mix it well. Measure the portions and serve.

Tips

Make sure that the rice has been thoroughly cooked to get the best taste.

I hope you have learned something from this book so far and would greatly appreciate it if you could leave an honest review on Amazon.com.

Meal Plan

Day 7

This is the final day of the meal plan. If you have managed to follow the meal plans so far, you should feel positive changes in your blood pressure.

Breakfast

For your breakfast, you can have the following meals.

1. A cup of whole grain oat rings cereal. You can team it with a medium sized banana and a cup of low-fat milk.

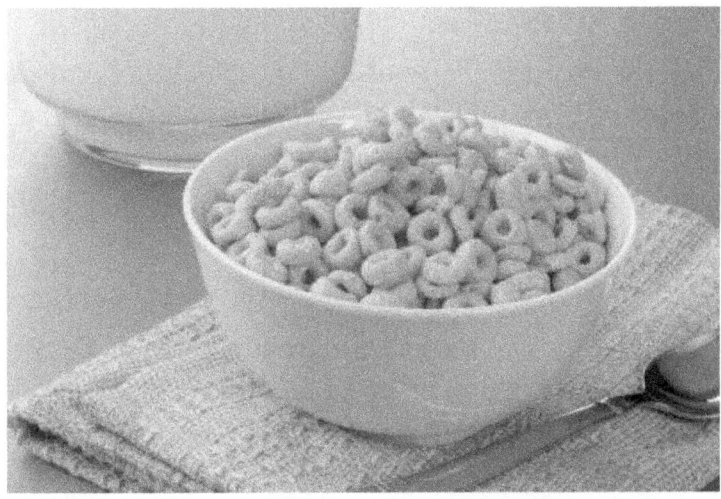

2. To wash the meal, drink a cup of fruit yogurt which is fat free.

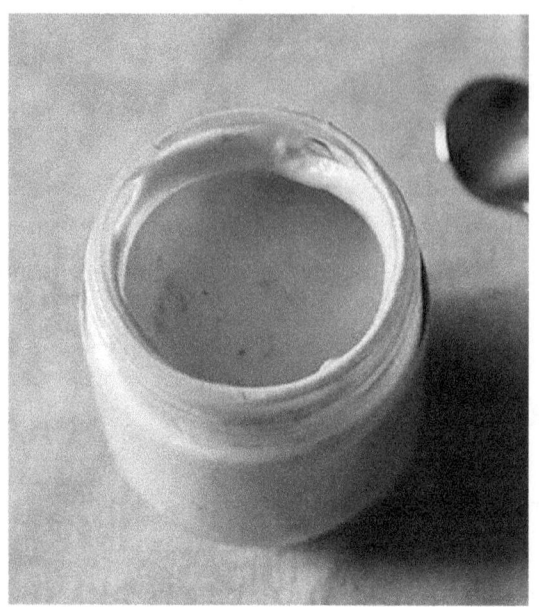

Tips

Try and ensure that the fruit yogurt which you consume is free of sugar. This will also help in cutting down the extra calories.

Lunch

The following meals look to be a great choice for DASH meal plan for lunch.

1. Tuna salad sandwich.

2. 1 medium sized apple.

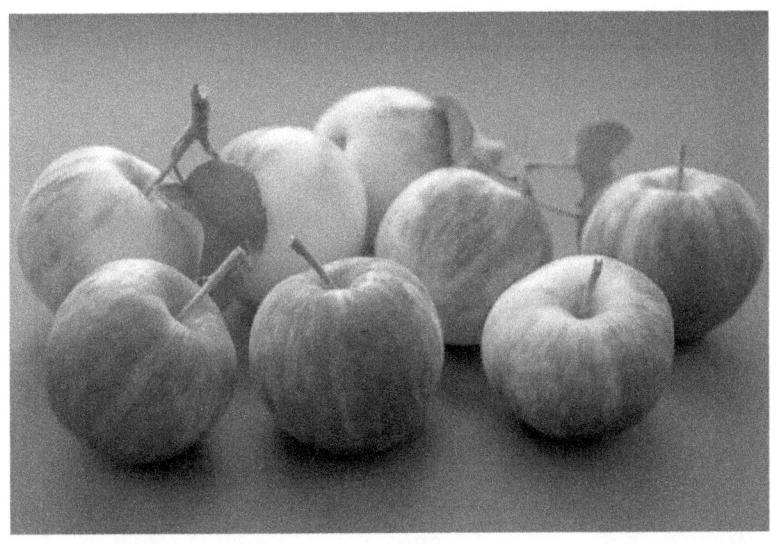

3. A cup of low-fat milk to wash down your sandwich.

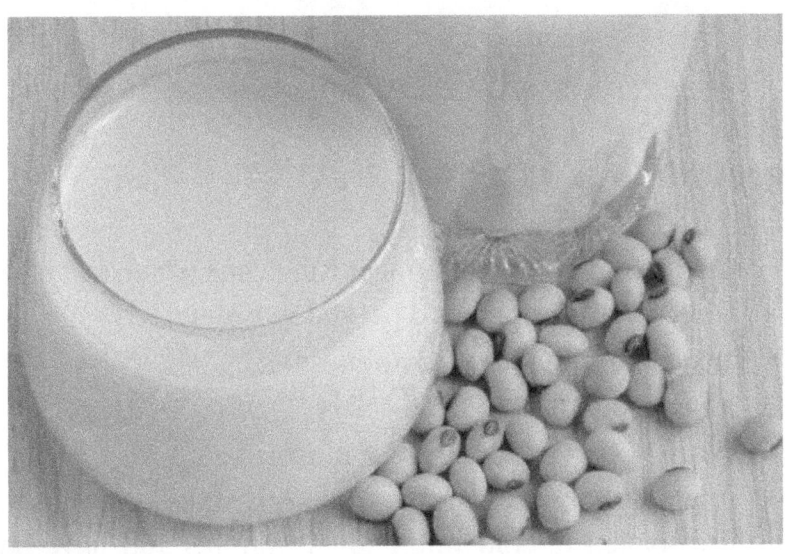

If you are looking for a recipe for tuna salad, here are the details.

Tuna Salad Sandwich

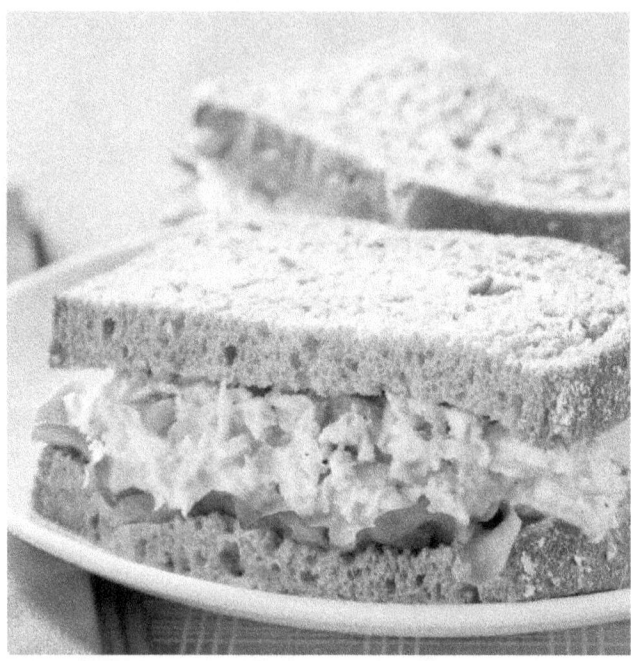

Ingredients

- Two 6 ounces of white meat tuna cans which have been thoroughly drained and packed in water.
- 1/3 cup of prepared mayonnaise.
- 2 tablespoons of minced celery.
- 1 tablespoon of whole grain mustard.
- 2 tablespoons of minced red onion. Make sure that they are soaked in cold water for 5 minutes and have been drained.
- Freshly ground black pepper.
- 1 teaspoon of minced parsley which has flat leaf.

Instructions

1. Take a small mixing bowl and break the tuna with the help of fork. Now toss celery, parsley and onion.

2. To this, add mustard and mayonnaise and season it with pepper. Store it to blend all ingredients thoroughly.

Dinner

This is the final meal in our DASH diet meal plan. To let your food buds have a delicious time, we are going to let you have finger licking lasagna for dinner. Let us take a look at the meals you can gorge upon.

1. 1/6 recipe zucchini lasagna.

2. A small whole wheat roll.

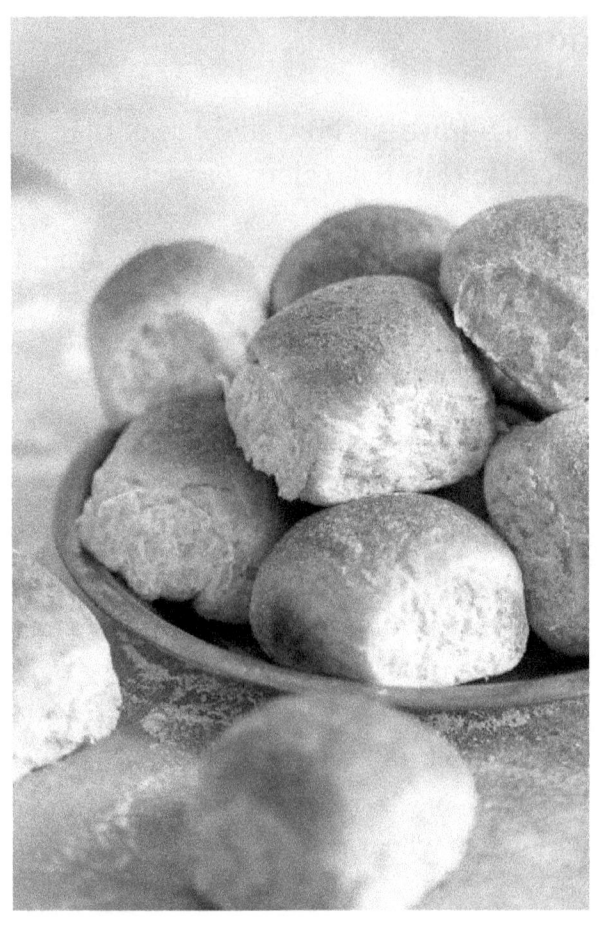

3. A cup of grape juice to supplement your liquid intake.

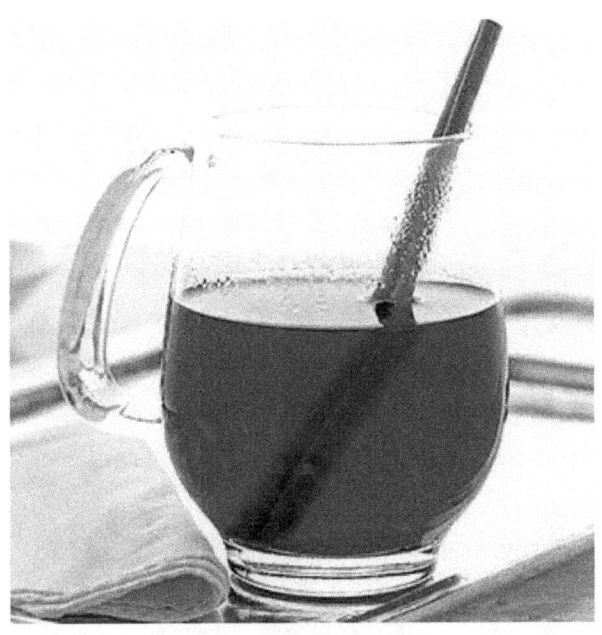

If you are looking to learn how to make zucchini lasagna, here are the details you need to follow.

Zucchini Lasagna

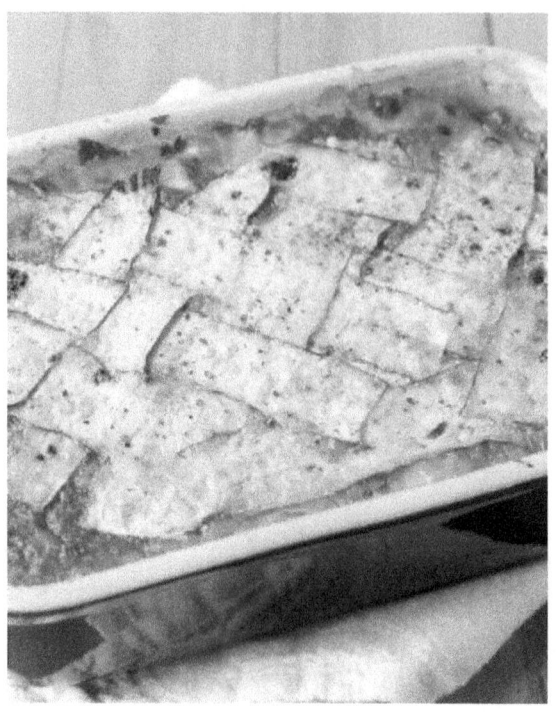

Ingredients

- ½ lb. of lasagna noodles. Make sure that they are cooked in unsalted water.
- 1 ½ cup of fat free cottage cheese.
- 1 ½ cup of sliced and raw zucchini.
- ¾ cup of grated, part-skim mozzarella cheese.
- ¼ cup of grated parmesan cheese.
- 2 ½ cups of tomato sauce with no salt added to it.
- 1 clove garlic.
- 2 teaspoons of dried basil.
- 1/8 teaspoon of black pepper.
- ¼ cup of chopped onion.
- 2 teaspoons of dried oregano.

Instructions

1. Preheat the oven to 350 degrees Fahrenheit. Take a 9 by 13-inch baking dish and spay it with vegetable oil spray. Take a small bowl and combine 1 tablespoon parmesan cheese and 1/8 cup of mozzarella.

2. Take another bowl and mix mozzarella and parmesan cheese along with the cottage cheese as well. Keep it aside. Now take tomato sauce and all other remaining ingredients.

3. On the bottom of the baking dish, spread a very thin layer of tomato sauce. Now, add a third of the noodles in a single layer.

4. Spread nearly half of the cottage cheese mixture above the layer of noodles. Add a layer of zucchini to it. Repeat the layering process and finally add a thin coating of sauce.

5. Top it with noodles, sauce and the cheese mixture. Cover the whole mix with an aluminum foil and bake it for nearly half an hour. Let it cool for 10 to 15 minutes and then serve.

Tip

In order to cut down the overall sodium content, you should make it a point to use unsalted cottage cheese.

If you feel like sharing the love and helping other readers decide if this is the right book for them, please take a few seconds to leave a short review on Amazon.com.

35 Fat-Blasting Tips

Tip #1 - Make a List

Ensure that you make a list of all the ingredients that you need for your diet. Most of us have the tendency to buy a lot of unhealthy ingredients like red meat and the likes when we go shopping without a list.

Once we buy them, it does not make sense to throw them away. Hence, we end up consuming them and therefore sort of cheat on our diet.

The purpose of making a list is lost here. The idea of having a list is to ensure that we are restricted by it. Make a list and follow it.

Tip #2 - Eat Before Shopping

Before you head out for shopping, ensure that you have a decent meal. You might wonder how going shopping on an empty stomach makes a difference.

Well, when we go shopping on an empty stomach, we end up picking quick fixes like crisps, chocolates and other processed foods to satisfy our hunger pangs.

These processed foods should ideally be the first things to go off your lists if you wish to control your hypertension. Moreover, it is really hard to focus on the plan in hand when you are hungry and you end up overstepping your control. Never forget to eat before shopping.

Tip #3 - Buy Fresh Vegetables

Buy lots of fresh vegetables when you go out shopping and include them in your recipes. Fresh vegetables are rich in fiber and are filled with anti-oxidants. You can begin by including these fresh vegetables in the form of salads. Ensure that there is always a green vegetable on your plate.

The best part about fresh vegetables is that they can be consumed even in large servings without having to worry about the implications. By consuming vegetables, you are ensuring that you are satisfying your appetite with foodstuffs that contains no saturated fat, which is generally a major contributing factor for hypertension.

Tip #4 - Read Labels

Often, we buy products without checking the ingredients and nutritional content on the label. These products can contain those ingredients which can induce hypertension. For instance, most of these packaged products and processed foods are high in salt content. The high salt content has a direct implication on one's blood pressure.

Increase in the salt intake can increase your blood pressure. Hence make it a point to read the labels of any foodstuff you wish to buy. You will actually be able to gauge how healthy these products are by just looking at the list of ingredients and nutritional content on the label and make a decision accordingly.

Tip #5 - Low Sodium

Pick only those ingredients that are low in sodium content. Often people confuse sodium with salt. Reducing sodium content is not about not seasoning your food with salt. It is about eliminating those foodstuffs that are high in sodium content. Processed foods are rich in sodium content and consuming them will increase your blood pressure drastically.

Eliminate processed foods from your diet and eat only those foods that are cooked naturally or minimally processed. Decreasing the sodium content can help in lowering the blood pressure. A good way to identify foodstuffs with low sodium content is to look at the labels given in the packages.

Tip #6 - Low Sugar

The DASH diet does not prescribe the complete elimination of sugar or sweets. It suggests the consumption of reduced amounts of sweets and sugar.

When you pick your desserts, ensure that they are low in fat. If you are someone with a sweet tooth, you can satisfy these cravings by using artificial sweeteners. These artificial sweeteners can help you regulate your sugar intake.

Make sure that you do not drink aerated drinks or flavored soda as they are packed with sugar which will add on to your calories intake in a day. Avoid including large quantities of sugar in your diet as they might lead to an increase in calories and your weight as a result.

Tip #7 - Eat Lots of Fruits

Include lots of fruits in your diet. Most fresh fruits are packed with fiber and anti-oxidants which will help you in maintaining your energy levels.

Include fresh fruits such as oranges, apples, bananas, dates, apricots and berries in your diet. These fruits are low in fat and hence they will not have a negative impact on your blood pressure even if consumed in excess.

If you are choosing frozen fruits, ensure that they don't have any added sugar. If you are opting for canned fruits, ensure that these fruits have been stored in their own juice as opposed to heavy and rich syrups.

Tip #8 - Vegetables, If Canned – No Sodium

As mentioned earlier, include lots of vegetables in your diet. If you are not able to get your hands-on fresh vegetables, you can opt for canned or frozen vegetables.

Many vegetables such as peas, tomatoes, carrots, spinach and broccoli come in both frozen as well as canned version.

If you are going for frozen vegetables, ensure that these do not contain any added salt or sauces or butter.

Similarly, if you are choosing canned vegetables, opt for those that are low in sodium content. The sodium content can be assessed by looking at the nutritional chart given on the cans.

Tip #9 - Whole Grains

Whole grains or cereals are a rich source of nutrients such as carbohydrates, proteins, fiber, vitamins and anti-inflammatory agents.

Regular consumption of these kinds of whole grains helps in lowering your blood pressure and also reduces the risk of various cardiovascular diseases.

Try to include whole grain varieties of bread in your diet such as bagels, pasta, pita, crackers etc.

These are also low in fat content. Ensure that the breads that you pick are low in sodium content as well by comparing the labels on their packages.

Tip #10 - Nuts, Seeds and Legumes

Legumes include beans, lentils, peas, peanuts and chickpeas. These are rich in carbohydrates, proteins, vitamins and fiber content.

Consumption of legumes helps in reducing the risk of contracting heart diseases and reducing the levels of blood pressure.

Nuts and seeds are also rich in proteins, vitamins, minerals and fiber. Nuts contain good unsaturated fats which help in regulating the levels of bad cholesterol in the blood.

These also help in reducing the blood pressure. Make sure that you do not include salted nuts in your diet as they can have the opposite effect.

Tip #11 - Cut Down on the Red Meat

Red meat comprises of pork, lamb and beef. Red meat is loaded with large quantities of saturated animal fat. Consumption of large quantities of red meat thus increases the amount of bad cholesterol in our blood and increases the blood pressure. It also increases the risk of developing cardiac related diseases.

Hence it is important that you lower your intake of red meat, if you are not able to eliminate them completely. You can easily regulate your blood pressure if your intake of red meat is considerably reduced.

You can perhaps have one serving of it every week. This way, the intake of saturated fat will not affect your blood pressure in a drastic way.

Tip #12 - Lean Meat, Poultry and Fish

An easier and healthier substitute to red meat can be either in the form of lean meat or poultry or fish. These have the same nutrients as red meat. In fact, these are healthier than red meat as they are devoid of high quantities of saturated animal fat.

Lean white meat includes turkey, chicken and other poultry. Consumption of certain kinds of white and oily fish can also lower the blood pressure. Make sure to select leaner cuts of meat always.

Tip #13 - Consume a Lot of Good Herbs and Condiments

Since your diet will be low in salt content, you can add flavor to your food by using herbs such as oregano, parsley, basil etc., spices, salsas, flavored vinegars and olive oil.

These seasonings help in adding a distinct flavor to your food. If you are going to pick the processed versions of these condiments, ensure that they are low in sodium content.

Tip #14 - Low Fat Dessert

When it comes to dessert, I have one suggestion; skip it. This will be absolutely possible for those of you who do not have a particular fancy for the sweet stuff.

Often what we see is that people eat some dessert after a meal simply out of habit or compulsion. That is a lot of unwanted empty calories that you are eating just for the heck of it. So, the next time, take the conscious effort to skip the sweet bowl.

For those of you with a sweet tooth, this advice may not be that easy to follow and hence I recommend that you consume low fat dessert. If it is just something sweet that you crave after a meal, then a piece of some sweet fruit ought to do the trick here.

The fruit need not be even a fresh one. For the purposes of a dessert, this can even be a canned fruit or a dry fruit.

Tip #15 - Use Half the Butter for Baking

Baking is one of those activities that consume a large amount of fat. That can be avoided if you exercise a little bit of caution. Based on what dish you are baking, check whether you can cut down on the amount of butter or oil being used. In many cases, a reduction of the oil will not amount to much of the taste being lost.

In any case, the target should be cooking the dish with half the butter that you will normally use. If you are able to cut it down by 30% or 35%, that itself is worth a lot.

Tip #16 - More Dairy Products

One of the fundamental principles of the DASH diet is the increased consumption of dairy products. This is because of the reason that in spite of what is commonly perceived of milk and milk products, they actually pack a punch in terms of nutrients.

Yes, it is a fact that they are also high in fat most of the times. But the nutritional value is something that is tough to ignore simply because of the fat content.

The solution is to completely shift towards consumption of low-fat dairy products. They contain the best of both worlds. On one hand you get all the goodness of milk and on the other you skip on the fat.

Tip #17 - Non-Stick Cookware

I believe that one of the most significant inventions that man has made in terms of kitchen articles is the non-stick cookware. They are truly wonderful things that can help you drastically bring down the amount of cooking oil or fat consumed.

Many a times, you are forced to use a lot of cooking butter or oil in order to facilitate the process of cooking rather than to increase the taste.

The non-stick frying pan negates this necessity. Hence as much as possible, make sure that all the cooking vessels in your kitchen have the non-stick coating on them so that you can go ahead and fry and sauté the onions without the accompanying guilt.

Tip #18 - Use Vegetable Steamers

Just like the non-stick cooking vessels, vegetable steamer insert is another brilliant invention that can help you cook the vegetables without any oil or butter.

These come in the form of inserts that can be positioned inside your saucepan. These fit into the bottom and let you cook the vegetables and greens without using even a drop of oil. But the catch is that when you purchase the steamer inserts, make sure that they fit flush with the cooking ware back in the kitchen. If not, the cooking process will not be uniform.

Tip #19 - Use the Garlic Press and Spice Mill

As we had mentioned earlier, Sodium is something that has to be kept away and used only in the bare minimum quantity necessary. I know that this also means that the food may lack in the taste area.

There is an easy and effective solution for this. Use more spices and garlic. These are items that will make even the blandest of dishes tasty.

And hence keep the garlic press and the spice mill handy and ready. If you feel that the dish lacks that zing, then give it a healthy dash of the spices and savor the difference.

Tip #20 - Fry without Oil

Now that sounds like an oxymoron, doesn't it? Well, the advancement in technology is so much that science has now made this possible. Yes, now you can fry without oil, or rather with a minute amount of oil. And this includes those deep-fried dishes as well.

This latest gadget for the kitchen makes it possible for you to fry those chicken legs or French fries or potato wedges with extremely less quantities of oil.

All that you need to do is slather a few drops oil on top of the dish and place it inside the device and voila!

Tip #21 - Make the Food More Spicy

As we had noted earlier, cooking food without much oil and salt may really drain it off any taste. What you can do is make use of a lot of spices and condiments that can add a lot of character to the dishes.

Be liberal with the use of black and white pepper. These are nature's treasure trove of nutrients and contain a large amount of anti-oxidants.

This way you are making the food tastier using ingredients that can actually be beneficial to your health. I agree that a lot of these spices and condiments can be a bit too pricey for your wallet, but then consider it money well spent for the betterment of your health.

Tip #22 - Rinse the Vegetable Well

It is one thing to consume more vegetables and greens as a part of turning towards a healthy diet pattern and it is another complete thing to be consuming some weapons grade chemicals in the form of insecticides and pesticides, just because the farmers got a bit trigger happy with the poison nozzle.

And the solution to this is as simple as it is effective. What you have to do is rinse the vegetables thoroughly at least 3 or 4 times before consumption. This is especially the case with leafy vegetables such as spinach that are more prone to insect attacks and hence are sprayed with more of the poison.

Tip #23 - Treat the Hunger Pangs with Salads

Now I understand that it is very hard to observe the restrictions imposed by a diet when the hunger pangs hit you.

Although the DASH diet is extremely lenient in terms of the food items that it allows you to consume, it will still be a difficult situation if the vending machine in your office has only the super-oily, super-sweet donuts.

In such cases, the best option for you will be a healthy salad. The best thing about salads is that they tick a lot of boxes. They are healthy, cost effective and only take a minute to prepare.

Tip #24 - Have a Lot of Soups

Soups are extremely good source of nutrients while at the same time being low in calories. They contain a huge amount of essential minerals and vitamins and can be considered as wonder foods in terms of the nutrient content.

And the best part about soups is that they are quite filling as well. It means a bowl of soup will make you feel full and satisfied and is hence a superb way of watching those calories.

But exercise caution when you order soup at a restaurant. Some of them may be notoriously high in salt content and hence will be completely inappropriate for consumption under the DASH diet.

Tip #25 - Keep Low Calorie Biscuits Handy

One of the best ways of avoiding the tendency to overeat during a meal time would be to keep snaking throughout the day at regular intervals. This keeps your stomach in a perpetually half full sensation and prevents you from hogging on the dinner table. To this effect the best option will be low calorie biscuits.

Always keep a pack handy with you. And make sure that they are not sweet cookies. It is important that the snacks should be low calorie, wheat or bran biscuits.

Tip #26 - No Soft Drinks

Well this is really unavoidable. When the ethos of the DASH diet is against sugar, then it will be an absolutely pointless thing to consume of-the-shelf soft drinks that are nothing but empty calories packaged in cans and bottles. Every form of soft drink that you find in the market today adheres to this formula.

An amazing alternative is to prepare your own homemade soft drink. And the best candidate for this is the good old lemonade or the lemon soda if you fancy a bit of fizz.

You can make them in the morning and carry them in normal bottles. The only catch here is this; make sure you make the lemonade or lemon soda with the minimal amount of sugar or salt.

Tip #27 - Be Adventurous With Your Cooking

Following any kind of diet may take a toll on you especially if your medical condition puts a lot of restrictions on the kind of food that you can have.

In case of people with hypertension, the food that you consume should be devoid of salt of excess oil or sugar. In such situations it is easy to be disgruntled with the rigors of your diet.

The best way to tackle this situation is to be as active and adventurous in the kitchen as possible. Make it a point to try out new recipes and dishes every now and then. This goes a long way in breaking the monotony.

Don't forget to share your thoughts on this book by leaving a review on Amazon.com. It takes just a few seconds.

Tip #28 - 4 Small Meals Instead of 3 Big Ones

This is one of those quintessential tips that come with every diet. In order to count the calories better and to keep the hunger pangs in check, one the most effective techniques is to eat 4 small meals that are spaced out accordingly instead of 3 big ones as breakfast, lunch and dinner.

This way the quantity of food consumed will also be less and you can make a bit of exception here and there by having something that is not exactly complying with your diet.

Tip #29 - Breakfast Like a King.....

Remember the old adage of how you should be eating breakfast like a king, lunch like a prince and dinner like a pauper? Well, that old saying holds true to this day.

Especially in case of the DASH diet!

The basic underlying principle is that that your food intake should be in ration with the energy spent by your body.

Tip #30 - Carry Food While Travelling

If you are of the kind who travels a lot, then it will be good idea to cultivate the habit of carrying your food with you in the course of your journeys.

Often the grub dished out by the airlines in the name if food can play havoc with your system. And it will be silly to expect them to prepare it the way you want your diet to be.

Tip #31 - Learn to Say No to Friends

When attending a party or during those office get-togethers, it will be a test of your resolve to stay away from all that pizza and burgers.

Especially, when your friends and colleagues are prodding you to take it easy just for a day and dig in to all that fried food. However, make the resolution to say a firm "No" to your friends.

Tip #32 - Space out Your Drinks

The teetotalers amongst you can skip over to the next Tip! However, those of you, who enjoy that occasional drink, need to pay attention. It will be a common situation for you then, where the urge to have that extra beer pulls at your heart in spite of your senses telling you to keep way from it.

The best solution in such situations will be consciously space your drinks so that you take an inordinately long time to finish the drink at hand. It takes a bit of practice to get this right but once you do, it will be worth it.

Tip #33 - Have Plenty of Water

Have plenty of water in a day to keep you sufficiently hydrated. Water has got a lot of beneficial properties that can really benefit you in a number of ways.

Among other advantages, sufficient intake of water ensures better fat metabolism in the liver. Since lower consumption of fat is one of the cornerstones of the DASH diet, drinking a good amount of water really helps here.

Tip #34 - Exercise

It is a fact universally accepted by researchers and experts that any kind of diet, including the DASH diet, works out to the highest level of efficacy when complimented by a healthy dose of exercise.

Some form or other of physical exercise is absolutely necessary to keep you fit and stimulate the body to make use of the nutrients that you consume through food.

Tip #35 - Eat in Moderation

I had saved the best for the last. Even the best and most nutrient rich food, if consumed in excess can land you in trouble. The ideal route is to consume food in moderation. Over time your body will get acclimatized to this routine and you will not have to make a conscious effort for this.

This means that you will feel full soon through the meal. There is an added advantage to this. Once you master this step and fine tune your eating habits, you can indulge in some of the dishes that may contain sugar or such other components.

Discover Scientifically-Proven "Shortcuts" & "Hacks" to Lose Weight FASTER (With Very Little Effort)

For this month only, you can get Linda's best-selling & most popular book absolutely free – *Weight Loss Secrets You NEED to Know.*

Get Your FREE Copy Here:
TopFitnessAdvice.com/Bonus

Discover scientifically-proven tips to help you lose weight faster and easier than ever before. With this book, readers were able to improve their weight loss results and fitness levels. So, it's highly recommended that you get this book, especially while it's free!

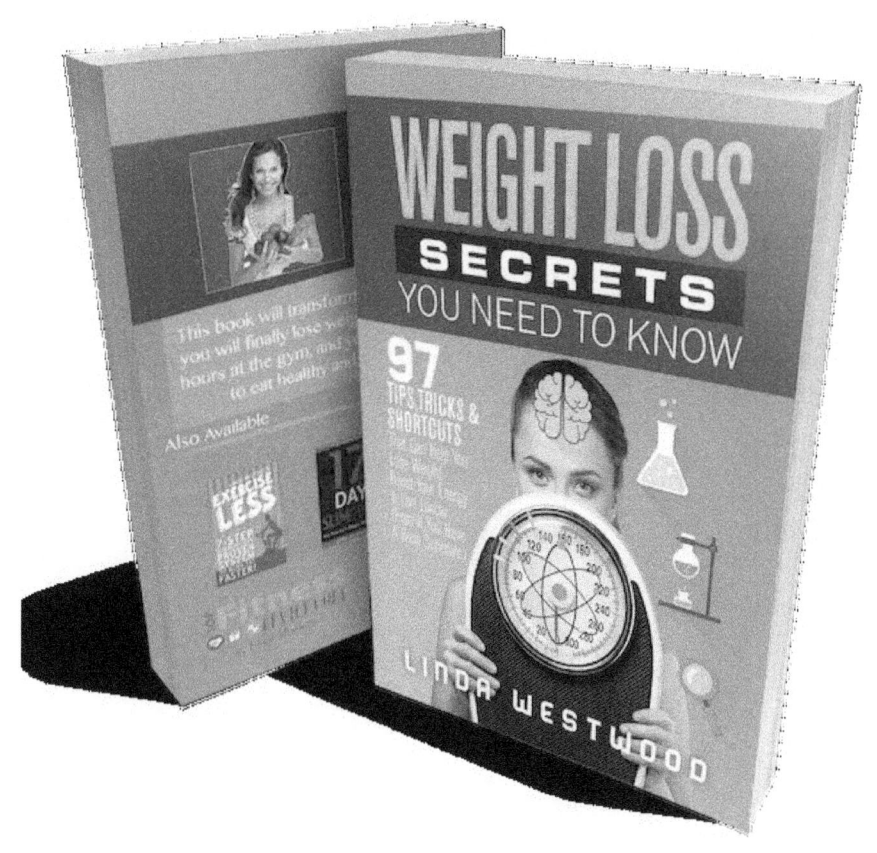

Get Your FREE Copy Here:

TopFitnessAdvice.com/Bonus

Final Words

I would like to thank you for purchasing my book and I hope I have been able to help you and educate you on something new.

If you have enjoyed this book and would like to share your positive thoughts, could you please take 30 seconds of your time to go back and give me a review on my Amazon book page.

I greatly appreciate seeing these reviews because it helps me share my hard work.

You can leave me a review on Amazon.com

Again, thank you and I wish you all the best!

Enjoying this book?

Check out my other best sellers!

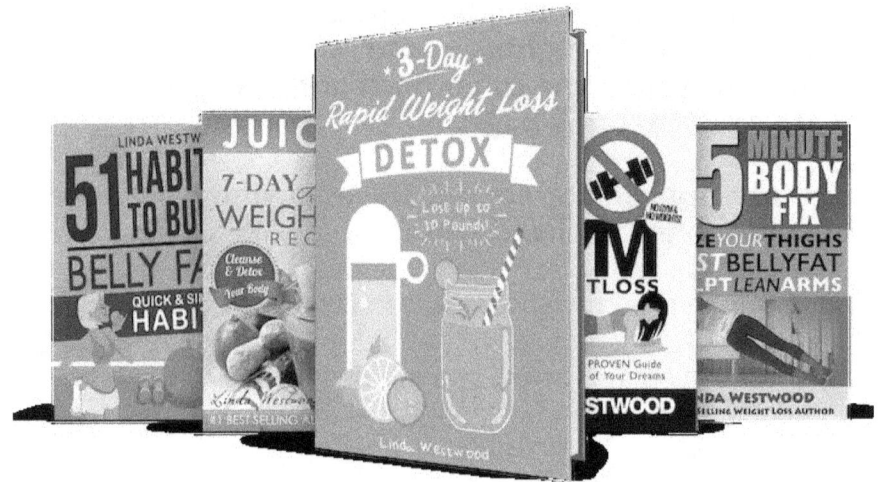

Get your next book on sale here:

TopFitnessAdvice.com/go/books

www.ingramcontent.com/pod-product-compliance
Lightning Source LLC
Chambersburg PA
CBHW031159020426
42333CB00013B/736